Contemporary Environments foi

HEMINGWAY NELSON ARCHITECTS
(Thompson Berwick Pratt)
R E C E I V E D
FEB 10 1994
Attention.............................
File.............................

MW01221681

Contemporary Environments for People with Dementia

Uriel Cohen and Kristen Day

Institute on Aging and Environment
School of Architecture and Urban Planning
University of Wisconsin–Milwaukee

The Johns Hopkins University Press
Baltimore and London

*In memory of Helen Bader, who dedicated her life
to the care of the elderly*

© 1993 The Johns Hopkins University Press
All rights reserved
Printed in the United States of America on acid-free paper

The Johns Hopkins University Press
2715 North Charles Street
Baltimore, Maryland 21218-4319
The Johns Hopkins Press Ltd., London

Photographs for part openings: page 2, Sidney Blatt; page 24, Ola Miller; page 176, Larry
Durkin. Photographs courtesy of Susan Gilster, Alois Alzheimer Center, Cincinnati, Ohio;
Altman Fleischer, photographer.

Library of Congress Cataloging-in-Publication Data
Cohen, Uriel.
  Contemporary environments for people with dementia / Uriel Cohen and Kristen Day.
    p.   cm.
  Includes bibliographical references and index.
  ISBN 0-8018-4489-4 (pbk. : alk. paper)
    1. Alzheimer's disease—Patients—Dwellings.   2. Senile dementia—Patients—Dwellings.
3. Long-term care facilities—Design and construction—Case studies.   4. Architecture—
Psychological aspects.   I. Day, Kristen.   II. Title.
    [DNLM: 1. Dementia.   2. Environment Design.   3. Facility Design and Construction.
WM 27.1 C678c]
RC523.C6523   1993
362.1′96831—dc20
DNLM/DLC
for Library of Congress
                                                                                                92-49834

Contents

Preface

Contemporary Environments for People with Dementia provides new design information to care providers, family caregivers, design professionals, and others interested in the creation of supportive and healthy environments for this population.

The potential field of design for dementia is increasing in scope. According to the Alzheimer's Association Public Policy Update of July 1991, "Over the past five years Alzheimer special care units in nursing facilities, adult care homes, and other residential settings have grown significantly. A 1989 report issued by the National Center for Health Services Research found 1,668 special Alzheimer units among the 22,604 facilities operating at that time. Of those, 3,112 facilities reported that they expected to open a special care unit by 1991."

Several recent publications have begun to provide design guidance and to explore relationships between the physical environment and behavior in this context (Calkins 1988; Cohen and Weisman 1991). *Contemporary Environments for People with Dementia* seeks to extend this design guidance and to provide information based on actual case studies—"real life" facilities that have implemented and experienced many of the design concepts and programmatic innovations promoted by design guides, researchers, and professional consultants.

Survey of "case studies" is a common, informal activity that takes place in almost every design project. Both client and designer visit and evaluate comparable places and programs, searching for insight, inspiration, and the latest information about ideas that work and those that have failed. *Contemporary Environments for People with Dementia* undertakes this task in a rigorous and systematic way and is organized to inform a multidisciplinary audience.

The physical settings occupied by people with dementia do not exist in isolation. They are an integral part of a large, complex system and are inextricably related to the social and organizational dimensions of this system. In recognition of this reality, *Contemporary Environments for People with Dementia* includes not only descriptions of architectural features but also of social and organizational aspects that relate—directly and indirectly—to the total environment of the larger system.

This book is organized in three chapters. Chapter 1 introduces the context of design for people with dementia. Chapter 2 describes and analyzes twenty case studies. Chapter 3 is an integrative analysis of selected key issues identified in the course of field work.

We hope that *Contemporary Environments for People with Dementia* will contribute to a more informed process of planning and design, ultimately resulting in enhanced quality of life for people with dementia and their caregivers.

Acknowledgments

The preparation and production of *Contemporary Environments for People with Dementia* involved the cooperation and support of many individuals, all of whom have contributed in important ways.

Primary support for the development of this book has come from the Retirement Research Foundation of Park Ridge, Illinois. Brian Hofland, vice president of the foundation, provided valuable input and continued encouragement of this line of research.

This project is the fifth in a series of research and development projects concerning environments for people with dementia conducted at the School of Architecture, University of Wisconsin-Milwaukee. The book is based on and is a natural continuation of prior work jointly conducted over four years with our colleague Gerald Weisman and other research team members. Part of the material in chapter 1 was adapted from past joint work and was written originally by Gerald Weisman, Keya Ray, and Barbara Cooper.

Powell Lawton and Polly Welch provided critical comments and constructive suggestions. Several experts in the field of design for dementia reviewed and commented upon earlier versions of chapter 3. The expert review by Margaret Calkins, Dorothy Coons, Sr. Edna Lonergan, and Susan Gilster, reinforced the relevance and validity of this chapter as the current thinking on specific characteristics of environments for this population.

Many individuals contributed their time and skills to this project. Dina Shehayeb and Hisham Gabr provided assistance with the handsome illustrations and graphic production. The Institute on Aging and Environment, the Department of Architecture, the Center for Architecture and Urban Planning Research, and the Graduate School of the University of Wisconsin-Milwaukee provided financial, organizational, and moral support.

Over the past two years, staff members, administrators, and architects involved in more than twenty settings cooperated with us, responded to our questions, hosted our visits, and provided not only the material on which this book is based but also insightful observations and suggestions based on their own personal experiences. Most of these people are listed in the respective sections of this book, and we express our gratitude to all of them. Without their cooperation, this project could not have materialized.

Contemporary Environments for People with Dementia

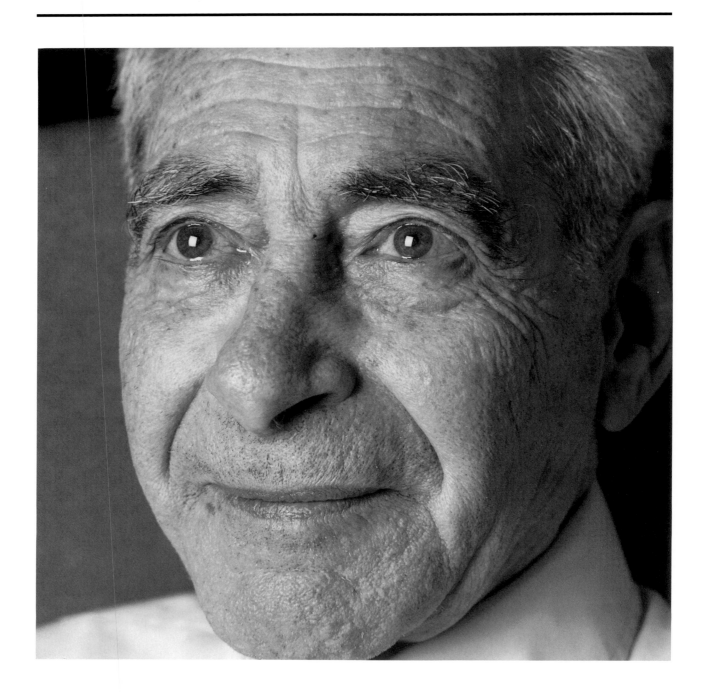

1 Introduction

This chapter describes briefly the basic problems and needs of people with dementia and their caregivers; the discussion places these problems in the context of the physical environment. It is followed by a list of principles for the design of environments responsive to this population. This chapter concludes with a discussion of the role of case studies in the design process and of the methods used in this case studies project.

People with Dementia

Although many readers will be familiar with Alzheimer's disease and its characteristics, some may find the following brief review a useful introduction to this topic. This section includes a description of the nature and history of the disease, current research topics, typical symptoms, and their effects.

- *Dementia* refers to a set of symptoms of various diseases and is not a result of normal aging.
- Alzheimer's disease usually develops after the mid-sixties, and the likelihood of developing it increases significantly in the seventies and eighties; however, the disease can occur earlier.
- More than 2.4 million U.S. citizens suffer from severe Alzheimer's disease.
- Of all residents of nursing homes, 60–70 percent suffer from some form of cognitive impairment, including Alzheimer's disease.

One of the most devastating illnesses associated with aging is Alzheimer's disease (AD). This progressive, irreversible neurological disorder is seen in its most severe form in 5 percent of the population over sixty-five years of age and in 20 percent of the population over eighty. Alzheimer's is the most common of the dementing diseases of elderly people, accounting for 50–60 percent of all such cases. In developed nations, it ranks fourth as a cause of death (after cardiovascular disease, cancer, and cerebrovascular disease) of elderly people.

The severe disabilities resulting from AD, which usually renders one helpless, are a major reason for institutionalization and have created a major public health problem. The magnitude of this problem is projected to increase as the number of elderly people in the population increases.

In the United States, the number of individuals with severe AD will more than double in the next thirty years (Heston and White 1983; Reisberg 1983; Lindeman 1984; U.S. Congress Office of Technology Assessment 1987).

Signs, symptoms, and prognosis

- Decline in functional, cognitive, emotional, and social abilities
- Reduced mastery and control over the environment
- Prognosis: people with Alzheimer's disease usually die seven to ten years after the onset of dementia, although this period may last up to twenty years.

The first sign of AD is forgetfulness, especially of recent events. Other cognitive functions are gradually compromised: judgment and the ability to orient oneself in space and to time are lost; new learning cannot take place; and expressive speech becomes difficult. Disabling personality changes and mood swings occur. This cognitive, emotional, and behavioral deterioration is not linear and may differ greatly among individuals.

Alzheimer's disease is relentless, irreversible, and devastating, as personal competence is eroded and the afflicted person slips into a state of complete dependence. In the final stages of the disease, which is eventually terminal, neuromuscular changes interfere with mobility and physical abilities (Heston and White 1983; Reisberg 1983; Gilleard 1984; Lindeman 1984; Shamoian 1984; U.S. Congress Office of Technology Assessment 1987).

Etiology

- Diagnosis is difficult.
- The cause is unknown.
- AD develops regardless of gender, race, or social status.

The etiology (or cause) of Alzheimer's disease is unknown. Early signs and symptoms may be mistaken for normal aging and, as the disease progresses, are difficult to distinguish from those of other dementias. Therefore, the goal of diagnosis is to rule out both other forms of irreversible dementia and other reversible dementias, which may respond to treatment. For this reason, a battery of tests, usually including a medical history, physical examination, psychological and laboratory tests, and various kinds of brain scan, may be administered (Heston and White 1983; Gubrium 1986; U.S. Congress Office of Technology Assessment 1987). Drugs are sometimes used to ameliorate symptoms such as agitation and paranoia, but, currently, no effective treatment can arrest the underlying pathological deterioration of AD.

Effect of dementia on caregivers

Most people with dementia are cared for at home, at least during the earlier stages of the disease (U.S. Congress Office of Technology Assessment 1987). The unrelenting demands placed upon the caregiver, usually the spouse or a close family member, create what Mace and Rabins (1981) characterized as the "thirty-six hour day" (1981). Without respite, the caregiver often becomes the second victim of the disease.

Problems in caregiving are exacerbated with the progression of AD and include difficulties with activities of daily living such as feeding oneself and getting dressed, getting lost or constant wandering, rummaging behavior, disorientation in time and space, agitation or occasional violent or catastrophic behavior, and withdrawal. The consequence of these problems is that eventually the person suffering from Alzheimer's disease cannot be left alone, and the care giver ultimately becomes bound to the home almost completely. Complete care is required at all times (Kelly 1984; U.S. Congress Office of Technology Assessment 1987).

Supportive therapies that help both the person with dementia and the family to adjust to the progressive decline by improving coping and daily living skills constitute the main assistance that can be offered. Activities and environmental modifications that help to minimize dysfunction and maximize remaining capabilities should also be implemented.

Linking Dementia and Environmental Design

Dementia and environmental design seem, at the outset, to be two very disparate topics; the relationship they bear to one another may initially be quite unclear. This introduction can provide only a brief examination of such an important issue. Understanding the relationship between architecture and dementia depends upon an understanding of three fundamental premises. First, it is essential to recognize that the role of the architectural environment need not be and should not be limited to the mere provision of physical shelter. Thoughtfully designed architectural environments represent potentially valuable, albeit typically underutilized, therapeutic resources in the care of people with dementia. Indeed, it has been argued that many of the behaviors attributed to dementia are, in part, a consequence of countertherapeutic settings (Coons 1985, 13). Both theoretical and empirical support for the *therapeutic potential of the physical setting* will be briefly reviewed.

Second, it must be recognized that the physical settings occupied by people with dementia do not exist in isolation; rather, they are integral parts of a larger, complex system and must operate in concert with the social and organizational dimensions of this larger system.

Finally, there is great value in enhancing the *residential* qualities of environments for people with dementia. Many such facilities, while well intentioned, do not, as a consequence of their medical or institutional characteristics, serve the best interests of people with dementia. To the extent possible, all therapeutic settings should retain the positive attributes of home.

The role of the architectural environment in therapeutic interventions for people with dementia has traditionally been quite limited. Interventions are defined and implemented in social and organizational terms, physical factors being limited to concerns of hygiene and/or esthetics. However, the study of the reciprocal relationships between people and their total environment over the past several decades demonstrates that the architectural environment is more than a background variable; it may exert a significant influence on behavior.

There are both empirical and theoretical reasons for efforts to utilize the therapeutic potential of the physical setting in the provision of care for people with dementia. Several studies assessing the influences of changes in the physical setting on people with dementia carried out by Lawton and associates are reviewed in Lawton (1981). A small-scale remodeling effort undertaken in a long-term care facility resulted in the creation of six single bedrooms plus adjacent semipublic spaces. Residents took advantage of this newfound opportunity for privacy and also increased the number of occasions on which they were observed outside of their bedrooms (Lawton, Liebowitz, and Charon 1970). In two pilot studies of the effect of environmental modifications on a psychiatric geriatric population (Fraser 1978), rearrangement of furnishings and introduction of materials for recreation and reading resulted in some social gains and a decrease in pathological behavior. In a pioneering demonstration and research project, Lawton, Fulcomer, and Kleban compared the behavior of severely impaired, elderly residents of a nursing home before and after transfer to new facility designed in response to their environmental needs (1984). Results indicate that, despite the expected decline in measures of basic competence, there was no corresponding decline in more pliable behavioral variables. "Even more remarkably, in five instances improvement occurred, and in only one instance was there a significant decline. This pattern of findings . . . confirms the presence of a clear prosthetic effect, to the point where the direction of a decline was reversed in some instances to become improvement" (p. 751). More recently, a longitudinal study of a special care unit conducted by Benson et al. indicated improvements in mental and emotional status and in basic functions of daily living twelve months after admission to the unit (1987).

A major research/demonstration project undertaken by the Institute of Gerontology at the University of Michigan created Wesley Hall, a special living unit for eleven people with severe memory loss (Coons 1985). Along with intensive training of the staff, a number of modifications were made in the physical setting; these included the introduction of softer and more domestic finishes and lighting and the provision of private rooms, a den, living room, a dining room, and a kitchen as part of the Wesley Hall unit. Staff observations indicated positive resident response to therapeutic interventions designed to reduce problem behaviors such as night wandering, incontinence, and combativeness.

Theoretical support may be seen as coming from several sources. The "environmental docility hypothesis" promulgated by Lawton and Nahemow (Lawton 1970; Lawton and Nahemow 1973) posited that "limitations in health, cognitive skills, ego strength, status, social role performance, or degree of cultural evolution will tend to heighten the docility of the person in the face of environmental constraints and influences" (Lawton 1970, 40). Thus, people with dementia, who often experience impairments of the kinds described by Lawton, may be particularly vulnerable to environmental influences. Conversely, even modest modifications in the environment which serve to reduce what Lawton and Nahemow characterized as the "press" or demand characteristics of the environment may yield significant improvements in both adaptive behavior and affect. At least some clinically based dementia research (e.g., Hall and Buckwalter 1986) emphasized the importance of conscious regulation of the demand characteristics of the environment, particularly in terms of sensory and social stimulation.

In summary, there is both empirical and theoretical support for the role of the physical setting in caring for people with dementia. Data suggest that modification of traditional room and unit layouts, along with complementary modifications in the organizational environment, can slow or in some cases even reverse the declines expected over time in the behavior of people with dementia. Such findings seem to be consistent with Lawton's "environmental docility hypothesis."

Guidelines for Planning and Design*

The following guidelines for the planning and design of environments for people with dementia are the product of an iterative process of development and are based upon the existing, albeit limited, literature on dementia and design, visits to actual facilities, and consultations with experts in the field. Given the newness of the field, the limited research, and the small number of significant demonstration projects, these guidelines are best viewed not as inflexible di-

*This section is adapted from G. Weisman, U. Cohen, K. Ray, and K. Day (1990), "Architectural Planning and Design for Dementia Care Units." In D. Coons (ed.), *Specialized Dementia Care Units.* Baltimore: Johns Hopkins University Press.

rectives, but as an effort to expand and stimulate thinking on the relationships between dementia and design; thus, they are hypotheses amenable to, and requiring, implementation and validation. These design and planning guidelines later serve as the basis by which the twenty case study facilities are analyzed (see under "Methodology", see chapter 2); in many instances, the observation of case study sites and interviews with facility administrators reaffirmed, or occasionally called into question the assumptions underlying these recommendations.

The following presentation of guidelines is organized in a clear hierarchy of environmental scale, from location and site concerns to micro-scale issues. Broad issues of philosophy, policy, and location are considered first. These are followed by principles that deal with environmental "characteristics" or "experiential qualities" and then principles for the overall spatial organization of settings. The final set of principles focuses on individual activity areas.

Only limited attention is directed to those architectural features—such as materials, finishes, and square footage allocations—most often associated with the relationship between the environment and human behavior. Although such variables may be quite important, their effects upon people with dementia are not always simple or direct; rather, their influences are through the contribution of features and general attributes of the environment, such as accessibility, stimulation, or privacy. Furthermore, such environmental attributes are typically most helpful in understanding and defining the therapeutic potential of physical settings.

Policy and planning decisions

The first sets of decisions to be made in the planning and design of environments for people with dementia are not fundamentally architectural in character; they are more clearly in the province of facility administrators and staff. However, their implications for the design of the physical setting are profound and pervasive. These key decisions are briefly reviewed here to ensure that they are consciously and carefully considered in the overall planning and design process and are not simply made by default.

Expanding the Continuum of Care

Residential options for people with dementia are typically conceptualized in terms of a small number of familiar environments: one's own home in the community, group homes, and long-term care facilities. It is critical to recognize, however, that what currently exists is not synonymous with what is possible. Indeed, some of the most creative and important approaches to the planning and design of settings demonstrate that new living options are both necessary and possible.

Environments for people with dementia are defined by the interaction of organizational factors (i.e., policy, program, and services), the social environment (e.g., formal and informal caregivers), and the physical setting. By combining these three subsystems in new and creative ways, it is possible to expand the continuum of care available to people with dementia. In long-term care facilities, for example, environments for people with dementia can be made less restrictive and more homelike. This approach might result in the deemphasis or elimination of the nursing station, the creation of more shared spaces for social contact, and reduced usage of hard, institutional materials and finishes such as tile, terrazzo, or vinyl.

Tapping Local Resources

It is essential to recognize that a setting that serves people with dementia is not an independent entity; rather, it exists in a larger environmental context that can provide important opportunities. Among the most important local resources are those family members and friends who may serve as informal caregivers and thus make significant contributions to the social environment of the setting. Decisions regarding the location of a facility can either strengthen or weaken such ties.

Proximity or easy access to specialized medical facilities can alleviate the need for the costly provision of these services within a residential setting. In addition to possible economic benefits, the removal of such services from an environment can serve to reduce its institutional or "medical" character and reinforce a more residential and familiar character.

Creating Small Groups of Residents

The transition from a small-scale residential environment to a large-scale group living situation can be stressful for anyone and is often especially so for people with dementia. New residents may be easily overwhelmed by a complex and unfamiliar environment (Peppard 1986) and may experience confusion, frustration, and feelings of helplessness. They are often removed from their everyday social support network of family and friends, as well as from the familiarity of their home, neighborhood, and, in some cases, community.

Such problems may be ameliorated by the creation of small groups of residents, at the scale of "family" as opposed to "institution." Group size in institutional settings is often defined solely in terms of the number of residents under the supervision of a staff member (e.g., the number of residents on a nursing unit in a traditional long-term care facility). However, it is possible to break such down functional groups into smaller social groups, often referred to as *households, families,* or *clusters.*

To emphasize further the concept of social groups, activity areas should be contiguous to a cluster of resident rooms. Such areas can then become the center of "household" activities, with these households functioning as self-contained units accommodating common functions such as dining. Staff to resident ratios need not necessarily be higher in such cluster arrangements than in typical "nursing units." Indeed, some authors and administrators have suggested that the creation of small groups of residents intensifies and enhances resident-staff member relationships and contributes to a staff perception of tasks as more manageable.

A variety of architectural strategies can be used to spatially reinforce the organization of residents into small groups. Shared spaces can be created for each such grouping; these spaces can serve traditional "dining room," "living room," or "kitchen" functions and can be so described and named.

General attributes of the environment

As emphasized in the introduction to this set of guidelines, one's experience of and behavior in a particular environment are often most strongly influenced not by specific architectural features or elements but by more general qualities or attributes of that setting. In the planning and design of environments for people with dementia, four such attributes seem to be particularly salient: image, negotiability, familiarity, and stimulation. In each case, it should be remembered that these attributes are a function not only of the physical environment but also of the interactions of physical, organizational, and social subsystems. Thus, the creation of a more "homelike" environment requires appropriate furnishings and finishes, patterns of ongoing behavior typical of those found in residential settings, and policies and programs supportive of such residential activities.

Noninstitutional Image

People with dementia are confronted with an ongoing series of changes in themselves and their world. Therefore, it is important, to the extent possible, to maintain their ties to that with which they are familiar and comfortable. A setting patterned after the outside community and its residential imagery—rather than after the medical model of the hospital and the conventional nursing home—can support people with dementia in retaining these ties to the healthy and familiar.

Breaking down the monolithic character typical of many hospitals and nursing homes is a necessary first step in creating environments more in keeping with the scale of human beings. Externally, this can be achieved by creating small, interconnected units as opposed to large, monolithic structures; internally, it can be achieved by breaking down the organizational as well as the physical structure of the environment (see under "Creating Small Groups of Residents [above]). Reduced use of institutional materials (e.g., ceramic tile, stainless steel), typically selected for their qualities of indestructibility, can reduce the institutional ambience; avoiding a totally uniform visual appearance throughout the facility may also contribute to this goal.

More Negotiable Environments

Although considerable attention in recent years has been directed to the creation of "barrier-free environments" (American National Standards Institute [ANSI] 1980), truly accessible or "negotiable" settings for people with dementia must respond to additional demands. Dementing illnesses may often exacerbate common, age-related problems in performing seemingly simple tasks, such as knitting, fastening buttons, or closing snaps. It may be equally difficult for people with dementia to utilize a variety of "control devices" in the microenvironment such as appliance dials, door handles, or telephones. Such difficulties reflect a variety of factors (Mace and Rabins 1981); these include apraxia (whereby messages from the brain may not be transmitted to hands and fingers), tremors, muscle weakness, and vision problems.

In addition to relatively familiar requirements for barrier-free design (ANSI 1980), a variety of strategies may be used to mitigate hazards and overcome barriers to negotiability in environments for people with dementia. Pastalan proposed the concept of redundant cueing, whereby the same information is presented via several sensory modalities (1979); for example, at the micro scale, light switches can be made conspicuous through color as well as form.

Objects in the microenvironment can often be designed with enhanced anthropometric fit to compensate for the decreased abilities (e.g., hand-eye coordination or visual acuity) of people with dementia. Examples would include lever-action handles instead of door knobs or pressure-plate light controls instead of common switches. Koncelik proposed self-correcting design of objects in the microenvironment (1976); such objects might include door locks with recessed tumblers to "guide" the key, thus directing and correcting the movements of people with dementia.

Things from the Past

Although people with dementia often cannot remember or be taught to remember recent events (Gwyther 1986), their long-term memory remains relatively intact until the later stages of the disease. Furthermore, the emotional components of memory may remain even after other components are lost (Coons 1985). The utilization of familiar objects—things from the past—can provide opportunities for the exercise and celebration of these remaining capabilities.

The use of things from the past can assist in the retention of ties to the healthy and familiar through the creation of more personalized and homelike environments, particularly for people newly relocated to residential facilities. Articles and events from the past provide people with dementia with the opportunity to reflect upon past experiences and environments (Rapelje, Papp, and Crawford 1981); such emotions and memories often serve to stimulate social interaction. In particular, the ability of residents to bring some of their own belongings and furniture to a setting can create a more familiar environment. Links to the past may be created in a variety of ways. Objects from the past may be interspersed throughout the public area of a special care unit or aggregated in a "museum" area.

Sensory Stimulation without Stress

Levels of sensory and social stimulation in environments for people with dementia may differ dramatically from those more commonly encountered in home environments. In some instances, there may be a virtual absence of stimulation characterized, for example, by monochromatic, repetitive spaces with little or no ongoing activity. In other cases, people with dementia may be bombarded by very high levels of stimulation including intercoms, alarms, or bright lights glaring on polished surfaces.

Attention must be paid, therefore, to regulating the character and intensity of stimulation in environments for people with dementia. The goal, in Mace's terms (1987), is "stimulation but not stress." Among the design strategies available for such regulation are two complementary approaches also employed for negotiability: amplification of the message and dampening of extraneous stimuli. Message amplification can be achieved by heightened contrast or redundant cueing, while dampening might include the use of sound absorbing materials, the elimination of intercoms, or the "painting out" of doors to service spaces.

Building organization

In contrast with preceding guidelines, this group of recommendations is largely "physical" in character, focusing on architectural rather than policy and program variables. Specifically, the common theme of these four guidelines is the arrangement of spaces relative to one another to provide areas for specialized activities, define levels of privacy, or ensure views to the exterior.

Family Clusters

Relocation to an institutional setting often presents people with dementia with major discontinuities in their social, organizational, and physical environments. Such transitions, and the overwhelming complexity and lack of familiarity they present, can be extremely stressful (Peppard 1986). Further confusion results when people with dementia are expected to carry out their normal patterns of behavior in a new setting to which they cannot easily relate. Therefore, it is important to create a physical and social environment that can aid in orienting people with dementia and in facilitating adjustment to their new environment. Moreover, the social structure of "family clusters" should be supported through the physical organization of spaces that accommodate the creation of independent territories for each family.

A necessary first step in the creation of such family clusters is the grouping or clustering of resident rooms. In addition to this, a rich mix of residential activities should be provided to emulate as closely as possible those found in homes, which will contribute to a greater degree of normalization. As well as providing opportunities for the full range of residential activities, the environment should allow a clear identification of different activity areas to help orient people with dementia. As found in most single-family homes, the activity areas for family clusters should be contiguous to the cluster of resident rooms. This would help define a public space at the scale of the family cluster for "household" activities.

Opportunities for Meaningful Wandering

Wandering is one of the many difficult behaviors attributed to people with dementia. Gilleard (1984) and Coons (1988) identified three types of wandering behavior most commonly found among people with dementia: (1) wandering as a consequence of disorientation, which may be as much a result of an illegible environment as of an incapacitated resident; (2) habitual activity stemming from previous experience; and (3) restless activity-seeking typically found in environments that provide very little to engage residents.

To reduce wandering from disorientation, design should ensure that the environment is easily read and that people do not get lost. Thus, repetitive modules should be avoided and memorable and unique landmarks should be introduced to provide residents with orientational cues that may help to reduce this type of wandering.

In recognition and acceptance of wandering as a habitual activity for some residents, walking paths should provide for more than mere physical exercise. Such paths should allow residents opportunities for passive involvement in activities without requiring them to participate, thus exposing them to social/sensory stimulation. Coons (1988) contended that, in a rich and supportive environment with numerous opportunities for involvement and participation, wandering behavior actually subsides.

Public to Private Realms

Oftentimes, environments for people with dementia do not provide sufficient variation in the levels of privacy available to residents. This is the result of organizational factors (e.g., staff members who do not knock and wait for permission before entering residents' rooms), architectural characteristics (e.g., large, undifferentiated dayrooms as the sole public or semipublic option), and combinations of the two (e.g., a policy that mandates and resultant design that offers only shared resident rooms). Providing opportunities along a gradient from public to private spaces offers residents control over the desired level of sensory stimulation, social interaction, and involvement in activities.

Facilities for people with dementia should provide spaces for solitude (such as private rooms and quiet nooks for one person), as well as for small group interaction (such as sitting areas separating each resident room from the rest of the household and small outdoor alcoves for private conversations). Many residents also suffer from understimulation and lack of socialization in large, impersonal, and sterile environments. Sociopetal (interaction-encouraging) spaces that are easily accessible to all residents and that are friendly and inviting in character are welcome public places in such facilities.

Positive Outdoor Spaces

Outdoor spaces can function as unique and relatively less expensive settings to meet a wide range of resident needs, providing variety and choice by allowing opportunities for both socializing and retreat within a safe and controlled environment. The outdoor environment is an excellent tool for enhancing a nonmedical, noninstitutional, positive image for people with dementia, staff members, and family. Such spaces also provide an important link with natural elements.

Wheelchair-accessible raised planting beds can provide residents with opportunities for gardening. Water features, such as pools, fountains, and waterfalls, located in well-landscaped outdoor spaces can offer visual, tactile, and auditory simulation, while places for pets might support links with the past. Outdoor spaces should be simple, be safe from physical and perceptual obstacles to movement and ambulation, and allow easy surveillance. Enclosures should be defined as unobtrusively as possible (e.g., plants, building mass) so as not to be either obvious or disturbing to residents. Recognizing the physical frailty of elderly patients with dementia, outdoor spaces should have a positive microclimate that ensures protection from excessive sun or harsh winds.

Large, undifferentiated, open spaces may be counterproductive and disorienting for people with dementia. Open spaces should be differentiated by alcoves, which can provide both settings for group activities and places for solitude and retreat. Such spaces might serve as interest points along an outdoor walking path, aid in spatial orientation, and assist in the creation of an outdoor environment with opportunities for a rich mix of activities.

Guidelines for activity areas

This final set of guidelines focuses on several of the most important spaces within a facility for people with dementia; these include entry areas, domestic kitchens, activity alcoves, resident rooms, common spaces, areas for bathing and toileting, places for visiting, and staff retreat areas.

Entry and Transition

The entry represents one's first impression of any facility for people with dementia. For this reason, it should be welcoming and noninstitutional in character. This can be achieved through the maintenance of residential materials and scale in the design of this space. The entrance and transition area should also function to decrease confusion and disorientation for visitors and residents. The design of an entrance and cloakroom that is removed from the sight of residents will limit interruption of ongoing activities by others entering or leaving the building. A disguised entrance storage area and cloakroom may also prevent residents from rummaging through their own and others' belongings and may decrease attempts to wander away from the unit or facility.

For the same reason, the entry represents an area where surveillance is desirable and necessary. Instead of disturbing alarm systems or humiliating "beeper" devices, surveillance can be sensitively provided by situating an administrative office where an employee can unobtrusively monitor coming and going from the unit or by introducing at the entrance technological devices that effectively prevent unsupervised exiting (such as doors that only open when the user simultaneously presses two nonadjacent buttons).

Domestic Kitchens

Domestic—small-scale, residential—kitchens in the home and in congregate living environments can provide for more than just essential food preparation.

Accessible and safe kitchen areas for use by people with dementia make available many meaningful and therapeutic activities and experiences, including such familiar household tasks as washing dishes, simple meal preparation, setting tables, sweeping, and folding towels. To facilitate this, the kitchen or kitchenette should be designed with plenty of seating and work space at small "kitchen" tables. The provision of a kitchen in a day care center or long-term care facility also enhances its domestic ambience, which can be further reinforced by the substitution of tile, wood, and bright, cheerful carpeting for stainless steel and high-gloss, monochromatic institutional surfaces.

The provision of a kitchen for use by people with dementia can reinforce the organization of a facility into small family "households." Its design should facilitate the kind of comfortable, informal socialization and reminiscence that often takes place at the family kitchen table. At the same time, the familiar kitchen "island" can function as an excellent point for informal surveillance of the facility by the care provider; this is a practical and noninstitutional alternative to the traditional nurses' station.

Of course, safety is a issue of some concern in kitchen environments. Ideally, these should be designed to allow maximum functioning for people at all stages of the disease without jeopardizing the safety of lower-functioning residents. All residents can certainly benefit from the provision of such a space; however, levels and types of participation in activities here may vary.

Activity Alcoves

Facilities for people with dementia often force residents to choose between very public spaces (e.g., large dayrooms) and very private spaces (i.e., their own bedrooms). Either of these extremes can be problematic. The presence of many other people in large, undifferentiated lounge areas may result in sensory and social overstimulation; these spaces likewise fail to provide that measure of privacy desired for interaction with family and friends. Retreat to one's bedroom may lead to confusion of day and night and may still (in semiprivate rooms) fail to provide desired levels of privacy.

Thus, the provision of a range of spaces from among which residents are able to choose can support interaction, privacy, and sense of control. Such spaces need not be large (a window bay is sufficient), but they should have some demarcation of their boundary (a railing, a change of flooring material) from the surrounding area. It is likewise desirable that these areas overlook ongoing activity, either indoors or out, and that they be situated along paths of movement, thus providing landmarks for orientation and places where wanderers might stop.

Residents' Rooms

In the single-family homes in which most Americans reside, the bedroom constitutes the most private region of the house, where the activities of sleeping, grooming, dressing, and bathing take place. In traditional long-term care facilities, however, resident rooms must serve as the setting for a broad range of public as well as private activities. The occupants of these rooms are forced to relinquish the right to privacy that most people take for granted. Also lost is the clear identification of function, which can prompt and support appropriate patterns of behavior. Therefore, in the planning and design of environments for people with dementia, attention must be paid to the traditional roles of the bedroom, as well as the elimination of conflicts between those functions that are relatively public and those that remain fundamentally private.

Common Areas for Each Family

In designing public areas within environments for people with dementia, the social structure of "family clusters" should be supported through the physical organization of spaces. The continuum of spaces should ideally range from the essentially private resident room to the shared public areas of activity within each family cluster. In the design of these common areas, one should bear in mind the goal of increasing social interaction among residents, as well as providing opportunities for individuality, privacy, and control.

One appropriate technique for establishing common areas involves the centralization of various activities at the core of each family cluster. This activity core becomes the public center of the cluster, much as the living room, dining room, and kitchen represent the core of family homes. Activity areas should be established adjacent to but not interrupted by circulation paths (Howell 1980). This strategy makes activities highly visible, thereby encouraging use, but does not force participation or lead to disruption. When possible, it is desirable to carve small subspaces out of large activity areas to create alcoves for passive participation or retreat, again in recognition of residents' need for privacy.

Finally, common areas should be roughly complementary to those found within homes, in terms of both scale and ambience. These domestic qualities will reinforce the residential nature of the space and highlight the ordinary activities of daily living, some of which might be as simple as food preparation in a small kitchenette or family activity around the dining room table.

Dining Areas

While there is no evidence to suggest that meals are as highly anticipated by people with dementia as they are by the general population, there is documentation that confirms the potential stress that can accompany this activity (Snyder 1984; Hiatt 1981; Roach 1984), often as a consequence of the loss of the ability to feed oneself and increased difficulty in the manipulation of utensils. Often, large, undifferentiated dining areas cause overstimulation—a consequence of too much noise and too many people—leading to agitation and confusion. Mealtimes, however, still serve as potentially meaningful social as well as nutritional activities. Maintenance of eating patterns developed over an individual's lifetime can provide continuity with the past and increase the scope for reminiscence.

Spatial organization that breaks dining spaces into separate subrooms or zones can reduce the institutional image associated with a large dining room that seats large numbers of people at long tables. Intimate dining areas with small tables seating family-sized groups of two to six people can evoke associations of home, increase comfort for residents, and reinforce manageability by staff. Noninstitutional furniture, together with a residential decor, can create a domestic ambience, deinstitutionalize the space, and evoke associations of "home."

Areas for Dignified Bathing

Bathing can be one of the most difficult activities performed by people with dementia and their caregivers. Because of physical deficits (including psycho-motor deficits that may affect the sense of balance) and decreased attention to personal grooming, the person with dementia often requires assistance in bathing or at least in getting into and out of the bathtub or shower; however, being lifted into a tub or shower can easily be an unsettling or even terrifying experience. In addition, the resident may resent the indignity of being assisted in bathing; many of the various institutional bathing devices (e.g., "cranes" or hydraulic lifts to hoist the resident into the tub) compound this indignity. These circumstances often combine to create a dislike of or an aversion to bathing in the person with dementia.

Bathing involves many potential threats to safety and security. The staff member may experience difficulty in lifting and maneuvering the person with dementia, especially problematic in the domestic setting, where the caregiver is likely to be an elderly spouse. Fear of falling during bathing or showering may increase aversion to bathing among people with dementia. Staff members in facilities for people with dementia are rightly concerned about minimizing the likelihood of falling in the bathing area. An additional safety concern is that unsupervised wandering into bathing areas may result in accidents. The design of bathing areas must respond to these valid concerns.

Whenever possible, people with dementia should be allowed and encouraged to take responsibility for those grooming activities (including bathing, whenever possible) that they can still accomplish with minimal stress or anxiety. Autonomy ought to be facilitated; for example, a resident may need assistance to use the bathtub but could possibly take a shower independently, seated on a nonslip chair in a shower with no lip and a downward sloping floor. In such a situation, independent showering may be a more attractive alternative to the resident; this opportunity should be provided.

Much of the equipment and many of the furnishings that have been developed to make bathing easier for the caregiver (e.g., hydraulic lifts and raised bathtubs) will probably seem strange to the person with dementia (indeed, to most people). Ideally, "bathing areas should be set up to be as reassuringly familiar and smoothly operational as possible. Bathing equipment that requires [people with dementia] to be suspended in unfamiliar contraptions" will likely be perceived as strange, threatening, and undignified (Hyde 1989, 39). In addition, noisy and crowded group bathing areas do not provide a calm setting or promote dignity for residents.

Aids to Independent Toileting

Although incontinence is a major problem for many people in the advanced stages of dementia, facilitating toileting can reduce the problem in the intermediate stages. Toileting areas should be easy to locate and identify and should be designed to be used independently by the person with dementia whenever possible.

Because of both the embarrassment of accidents and the need for assistance from others, toileting may become a less than private and dignified activity. Even upon locating the toilet area, people with dementia may have difficulty using these facilities independently because of problems of limited access or difficulty in entering and using the facilities without assistance. Incontinence becomes a major problem in the advanced stages of dementia in terms of sanitation, loss of dignity, and associated stigmatization.

Incontinence is quite problematic for staff members in any type of facility for people with dementia, necessitating extra time and effort in caregiving and clean-up. In addition, assisting people with dementia in locating, identifying, and using toileting facilities is time consuming for both professional and family caregivers.

The self-esteem and dignity of the person with dementia may be closely associated with autonomy and the preservation of privacy and independence in toileting. To bolster independent use of toileting facilities, one must increase the visibility of these areas to people with dementia and explore alternative means of enhancing residents' awareness of the need to use such facilities. Whenever possible, facilities for people with dementia should maintain the familiar appearance and usage of toileting areas and should avoid alternatives that invade residents' privacy (e.g., group toileting areas) or that obscure the intended use of the areas (e.g., a powder room or lounge area in a public restroom may obscure the function of the space for some residents).

Places for Visiting

Visitation from family and friends is an important component in the lives of people residing in facilities for people with dementia. It is therefore important for these facilities to provide spaces for visiting other than resident rooms, crowded dayrooms, or corridors that do not readily accommodate such activities. It is reasonable to assume that, at least in the early stages of the disease, residents might benefit from environments that offer opportunities for relatively private conversations. Environments supportive of visitors' needs might encourage more frequent visits, which could prove beneficial to people with dementia and family staff and members. To this end, residents and their visitors should have the opportunity to meet and converse in small and intimate settings.

Persons with dementia may become passive. Visiting them often becomes a very frustrating experience for family members, who might find conversation difficult. Spaces for visiting might remedy this situation by including things from the past to serve as catalysts for conversation with people with dementia, whose long-term memory may be relatively intact. It would also be useful for such spaces to offer "something to do." Places for visiting might establish links to the outside, enabling visitors to take a walk with a resident, or could provide some simple games that residents and visitors might play together.

Retreat Areas for Staff Members

Care for people with dementia is an extremely demanding and draining job, from which staff members will need an occasional break. In addition, some of the tasks involved in this job require a place where activities such as charting and private conversations with physicians and colleagues can take place without interruption from residents or visitors. Environments for people with dementia should include a space (or spaces) for staff retreat, work task completion, private conversation, socialization, and decompression. These places can also serve as the location for any dangerous equipment or supplies (e.g., hot plate, coffee pot, medication) or personal items (staff members' purses and coats) that should be kept from the person with dementia.

To meet these needs, staff retreat areas should provide comfortable seating, sufficient storage space, and a convenient work area for those who will use it. In addition to a break area and work space, the staff retreat area may serve as a resource, training, and information center for staff members by including such items as journals, staff mailboxes, and a bulletin board with postings of policy changes and upcoming events. The staff retreat area should be accessible to staff members and yet out of the path of residents. The design of such a place should reinforce the residential image of the environment, and staff members' perception of themselves as valuable people. Staff members' access to a private place for temporary retreat in the facility can increase the quality of life and of care giving for both employees and residents.

A final note concerning design principles: the behavior of people with dementia—and their needs—change significantly over the course of the disease. The application and use of the design principles listed above must take this fact into consideration, as particular modifications may be more or less appropriate for people in various stages.

The Role of Case Studies in the Design Process

The design or renovation of facilities for people with dementia is a complex process. Informed programming and design are critical prerequisites for successful resolution of all key goals and issues. Care providers and facility planners must have a clear understanding of the particular environmental needs of people with dementia, as well as the needs of their caregivers. Equally important are the knowledge of applicable design principles and concepts; the range of environments currently available for this user group; innovations and

Figure 1.1

Informed programming and design. A schematic diagram of the development process.

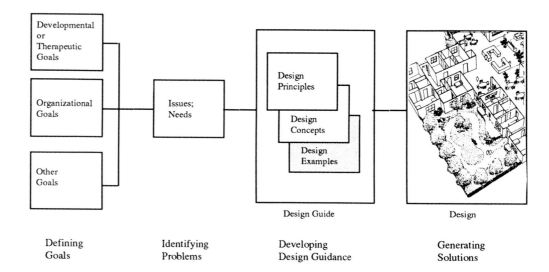

Developmental or Therapeutic Goals			
Organizational Goals	Issues; Needs	Design Principles / Design Concepts / Design Examples	Design
Other Goals		Design Guide	

| Defining Goals | Identifying Problems | Developing Design Guidance | Generating Solutions |

emerging trends in this domain; and the latest information about what "works" and "doesn't work" and for whom.

An informed programming process has four phases: defining goals, identifying problems, developing design guidance, and generating solutions (Fig. 1.1).

Design examples—case studies—are an integral part of the "design guidance" phase and serve as a companion to the design guide. Because the programming and design processes are cyclical rather than linear, case studies offer critical input for other phases as well—shaping goals, assisting in problem identification, and pointing toward possible design solutions.

Case studies are an important source of information for preprogramming, programming, and design of facilities. Visiting selected, exemplary settings is a common first step in the design process for both clients and designers of facilities.

The use of the "case study method" is practiced by professionals in a variety of ways: most often, it takes the form of informal, personal site visits. Sometimes, however, case study research is a more systematic process, documented and accompanied by a review of published case studies (e.g., articles in journals and books that are primarily dedicated to case study descriptions and analysis).

The potential of case studies to inform the design process depends on their quantitative and qualitative features: however, even informal and casual study of a small sample of sites can yield useful information and shed light on all parts of the process, answering questions such as What are the typical goals of the case study sites? What are common—and uncommon—problems? What are the design principles and design concepts most valued and most often applied? How do facilities resolve all of the above through design?

Many lessons and experiences can be shared and may be adopted as either proven, tested solutions or, more importantly, as catalysts for innovation and experimentation.

Methodology

The systematic and rigorous process of this study required the development of formal criteria for description and evaluation of settings and the employment of several techniques for gathering and handling information.

Selection of the sample of case studies

Although the number of special care facilities for people with Alzheimer's disease is growing, the definition and classification of these environments is not standardized. Available data indicate great variation in philosophy, policy, and design among facilities that consider themselves as providers of special care for this population (Ohta and Ohta 1988; Mathew et al. 1988).

The intent of this study was to include settings that represent diversity on several dimensions:

- facility type, including day care and respite care centers, group homes, long-term care facilities, and innovative continuum of care settings;
- operational diversity, including facilities that accommodate both service and research and demonstration;
- rural, suburban, and urban settings;
- both newly designed and renovated buildings;
- facilities that have played an important, historical role in promoting advances in environments for people with dementia.

The pool of candidate sites from which to select case study settings was generated through experts' recommendations, review of the literature in this field, and the authors' own familiarity with particular projects. The final selection was influenced primarily by the criteria described above.

The sample is not exhaustive, nor is it a representative cross section of current case options. Rather, the sample of case studies is used to highlight new trends, introduce new ideas and useful concepts, and examine strengths and weaknesses of various design, organizational, and policy solutions. Therefore, the inclusion of facilities in this report should not be construed as endorsement of these places, nor are these facilities suggested as "ideal," prototypical environments.

Types of analysis

The information gathered and presented in this book falls under two broad categories: description and critical analysis. Both types of information were gathered and generated in a systematic and structured process to ensure comprehensive coverage, comparability, and consistency.

Four primary activities—and related research instruments—were employed:

1. Description of facilities: A standardized survey questionnaire was developed to gather factual information about each setting. The questionnaire covered various aspects of the setting—environmental design, history and development, organization, operation, and activities. This survey instrument was used during the site visits and in selected cases was completed by the facility's staff.

2. Evaluation of performance: Site visits included interviews with staff members and administrators. The formal survey included several evaluative ques-

tions about positive and negative experiences and other personal reflections about design for dementia.

3. Criteria-based assessment: All settings—including those in the design stage—were reviewed by the authors against a standardized list of design principles (see under "Guidelines for Planning and Design, above). The design principles were adopted from the design guide *Holding on to Home* (Cohen and Weisman 1991). Notable applications, as well as major omissions, were listed and described in each site.

4. Survey of experts' opinions: Chapter 3 is organized as an integrative analysis of major issues and topics of interest. A number of these issues remain controversial among researchers; others have no consensus among practicing professionals. A draft of the chapter was circulated for review among several experts in the field to gather additional information and comment, which are incorporated in the chapter.

The methods and types of analysis are reflected in the organization of the book. Chapter 2 includes the descriptive information about each setting. The third page of each description includes a criteria-based assessment reflecting upon the design of the facility, with positive and negative aspects demarcated by + and − symbols, respectively, in the margin of each annotation. Chapter 3 includes a discussion of key issues identified as important topics in the course of field work, supplemented by experts' opinions.

A great deal of the information in this book—such as basic concepts and innovations—is not time dependent, but several items are temporal in nature. Costs, the nature of activity programs, and even the organization of the physical environment do change with time.

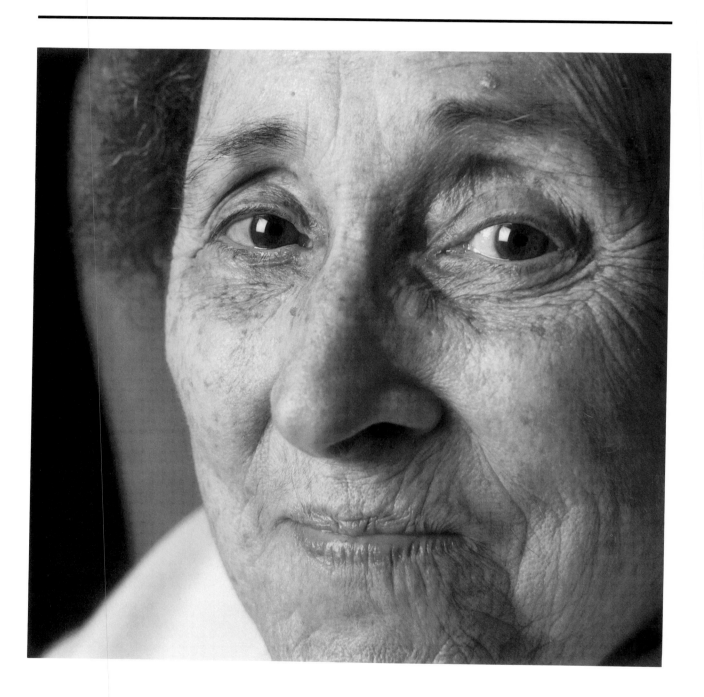

2   Case Studies

This chapter includes descriptions and analyses of selected case studies of environments for people with dementia (see table 2.1). The sample is not exhaustive, nor is it a representative cross section of current care options. Rather, as described in chapter 1, the sample of case studies is used to highlight new trends, introduce new ideas and useful concepts, and examine strengths and weaknesses of various design, organizational, and policy decisions. Therefore, the inclusion of facilities in this chapter should not be construed as endorsement of these places, nor are these facilities suggested as "ideal," prototypical environments. In addition to the primary case studies, we include brief case studies of facilities that are still unbuilt or that serve as useful demonstrations of selected key points.

Table 2.1 Case Studies Identified by Key Physical and Organizational Characteristics

	Facility/Service Type				Physical and Operational Status	
	Day Care	Respite Care	Group Home	Long Term	Free-standing Independent	Affiliated with Other Facilities
Alois Alzheimer Center, Cincinnati, OH	●	●		●	●	
Alzheimer's Care Center, Gardiner, ME	●					●
Alzheimer's Disease Residential Center, San Francisco, CA	●			●		●
Corinne Dolan Alzheimer Center at Heather Hill, Chardon, OH	●	●		●		●
Friendship House, Cedar Lake Home Campus, West Bend, WI	●			●		●
Minna Murra Lodge, Queensland, Australia			●		●	
New Perspectives Group Home #4, Mequon, WI			●		●	
Pathways Project, MJHHA, Miami, FL	●	●	●	●		●
St. Ann Day Care Center, St. Francis, WI	●					●
Therapeutic Garden, Sunset Haven, Niagara, Ontario, Canada				●	—	—
Weiss Institute, Philadelphia Geriatric Center, Philadelphia, PA				●		●
Woodside Place, Oakmont, PA				●		●
Alexian Village, Milwaukee, WI				●		●
Cedar Acres Adult Day Center, Janesville, WI	●					●
Elderkare, Beloit, WI			●	●	●	
Hale Kako'O, Honolulu, HI	●	●			●	
Helen Bader Center, Milwaukee Jewish Home, Milwaukee, WI			●	●		●
John Douglas French Center, Los Alamitos, CA	●	●		●	●	
Namesté Alzheimer Center, Colorado Springs, CO				●	●	
Stonefield Home, Middleton, WI			●		●	

| Design and Construction | | Physical Setting | | | Private/Public Sector | | Type of Licensure | | | | |
New	Renova-tion	Rural	Suburban	Urban	Profit	Non-Profit	Skilled Nursing Facility (SNF)	Assisted Living/ Rest Home	Boarding Care	Group Home (CBRF)	Day Care
	•		•		•		•				
•		•				•			•		
	•			•		•		•			•
•		•				•		•			
•		•				•	•				
•			•			•				•	
•			•		•					•	
•			•			•	•	•	•	•	•
	•			•		•					•
	•		•			•	—	—	—	—	—
•				•		•	•				
•			•		•				•		
•			•			•					
	•	•				•					•
•			•		•					•	
•				•		•					•
•				•		•				•	
•				•	•		•				
•			•			•	•				
•			•		•					•	

Alois Alzheimer Center

Address	70 Damon Road Cincinnati, OH 45218 (513) 825-2255
Owner	Jonas-Cory, Inc.
Staff contact	Susan Gilster, Executive Director
Facility type	Freestanding, licensed nursing home, with long-term, day, and respite care
Residents	82 nursing home residents, with up to 5 day care and respite clients
Staff	94 full- and part-time staff members, including an executive director, executive assistant, director of social service, director of recreation and activities, activity assistants, director of nursing, R.N.s, L.P.N.s, a medical records clerk, nursing assistants and orderlies, an office manager and receptionists, and housekeeping, maintenance, and dietary personnel
Staff to resident ratio	1:5 from 7:00 a.m. to 3:00 p.m.; 1:6 from 3:00 p.m. to 11:00 p.m.; 1:10 from 11:00 p.m. to 7:00 a.m.
Site/context	The single-story facility site is located on seven acres of land in a residential neighborhood, accessible to major thoroughfares and surrounded by preserved national woods. The building is a former school converted to assisted living and then renovated into its present use.
Size	27,000 square feet (approximate)
Date of completion	Opened May 1, 1987
Architects	Unknown
Publications	(1991). The emergence of special care units. *Journal of Long-Term Care Administration,* Spring. (1991). Developing a viable residence for persons with Alzheimer's disease. *American Journal of Alzheimer's Care and Related Disorders and Research,* January/February. (1991). Developing the first Alzheimer facility in the United States. In *Carers, professionals, and Alzheimer's disease.* London: John Libbey and Co.

This analysis is based largely on staff self-reports.

Figure 2.1   **Plan of the Alois Alzheimer Center, Cincinnati, Ohio.**

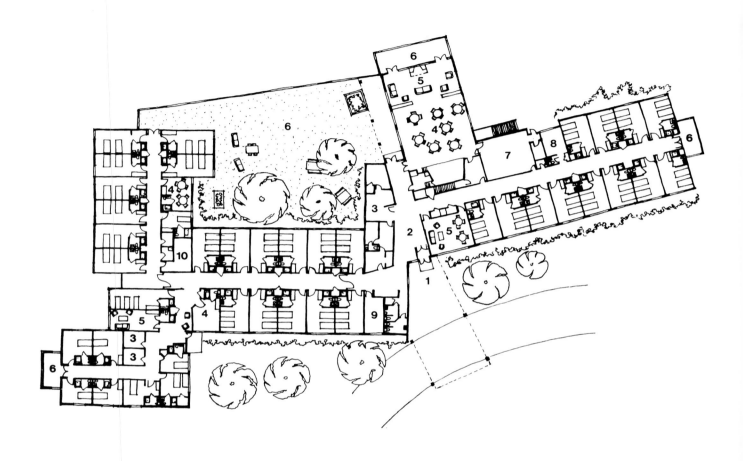

1   entry
2   lobby
3   administration
4   dining/activity room
5   living rooms
6   secure courtyards
7   kitchen
8   staff retreat
9   beauty shop
10   bathing area

Responding to Change

− The floor plan of the facility is a product of successive renovations from a school, to an assisted living facility, to its current use. It represents a very conventional physical organization of a long-term care facility, with typical, double-loaded, long corridors.

+ Despite the restriction of the physical structure, the staff continually adapts and changes the program and the use of space to respond to changing needs and emerging trends. For example, a number of residential rooms were converted to satellite dining rooms and social spaces when residents' needs demanded more space for small-scale social interaction.

Small Groups of Residents

+ The building is divided into three residential clusters. This division—both physical and programmatic—permits residents to participate in the least restrictive environment possible. Each cluster has its own dining and social/activity spaces.

Continuum of Care

+ The building represents a comprehensive continuum of specialized care: in addition to day care and short-term respite care, the three residential clusters accommodate persons grouped by functional and cognitive abilities, as well as by individual needs and desires.

Positive Outdoor Space

+ The pastoral setting contributes to a tranquil atmosphere; the primary courtyard is large and secure and includes a variety of features such as a planter, seating, and an adequate path.

Noninstitutional Image

+ Despite the institutional building type, there is great effort to reinforce a residential and domestic ambience through interior design and finishes and through programming.

− Ironically, the traffic generated by a large number of staff members, researchers, and administrators and the numerous programs taking place in the building, may compromise residential intimacy.

Circulation and Wandering

− Because of the original, institutional floor plan, the public circulation is limited to a double-loaded corridor originating in a public lobby. Despite the domestic furnishing and finishes, walking in the corridors does not provide an ideal meaningful wandering experience; the major intersection in the lobby near the entrance represents a potential for agitation and security problems.

Background
History

The Alois Alzheimer Center is a single-story, freestanding facility dedicated exclusively to the care and study of individuals with Alzheimer's disease and dementia. It is located in Greenhills, a small residential area in a northwest suburb of Cincinnati, Ohio. The facility originally served as an elementary school building, which was abandoned in the early 1980s because of declining school enrollment. Before becoming the Alois Alzheimer Center, the school was renovated to be an assisted living complex. It was selected for development as a specialized dementia facility in part because of its removed location and quiet, natural, low-stimulus surroundings.

The process of development

The center was developed following experience with cognitively impaired individuals in traditional environments. Consultation with local gerontologists and national experts confirmed the need for a specialized environment that addressed the needs of people with dementia. In June 1986, the state of Ohio passed legislation that allocated a limited number of specialized nursing home beds for this population.

The center is designed to provide a continuum of care within one setting, offering adult day care and respite care, as well as residential care to individuals at all stages of the disease. It has continued to change and evolve with experience and in response to the decline of the resident population.

Mission

The facility was specifically intended to improve upon traditional models of care by directing all efforts toward meeting the needs of people with cognitive impairment, specifically those with Alzheimer's disease, through an environment and program designed to improve the quality of life for both residents and family members.

Funding

Initial funding for the development of the center came from the organization's own resources. Ongoing support is provided by private residential funds and insurance claims. Educational programs are self-sustaining, and much of the research is supported by research grants.

Costs

Self-pay residents are charged $90 to $110 per day, based on the level of care and staff assistance required. Individual residents are evaluated using a modified Haycox Dementia Rating Scale, and fees are assessed on this basis. All residents are reassessed on a quarterly basis, and rates are adjusted accordingly. Administrators note that it is not unusual to experience a rate decrease after admission to the center, as individual function frequently improves following placement. (An informal survey conducted by the center demonstrated that other, nonspecialized local facilities providing skilled care range in price from $82 to $175 a day.) Private and semiprivate room rates are identical.

Respite care residents are assessed utilizing the same information as for permanent residents, with an additional charge of $2.50 per day added to the base rate.

Day care participants pay $40 per day (for approximately eight hours) or $20 per half day, including meals and snacks.

The facility is currently meeting and exceeding expenses; however, initial investment debt remains. Expectations are that this debt will be eliminated within the next few years.

<table>
<tr><td>*Services*</td><td>

Residential Care

The facility was developed to provide a continuum of care to individuals with Alzheimer's disease and dementia at any stage, from the early stages through the end of life.

Day Care

The day care program was developed to benefit participants by providing an environment in which they could achieve and succeed, meet new friends, remain active, and participate in life, as well as to provide support for families. The day care program can accommodate up to five participants at a time and offers full and half-day services. Hours are flexible to meet the needs of participants and families. Participants are encouraged to attend day care at least two days per week initially or more if necessary while becoming adjusted to the program. The day care was slow to develop but now has an average of three to five participants a day.

Day care participants receive meals and snacks and may receive assistance with personal care if individually arranged, in addition to individualized programming and recreational activities. Other services available at the center are negotiated individually, such as beautician services, podiatry, and dentistry.

Respite Care

The respite care program was developed to assist participants and families providing care at home. It has been quite helpful to families in time of crisis and is also utilized as a "test" to determine participants' and families' reaction to the center before long-term placement.

Numerous families make use of respite care several times a year to meet their individual needs for holiday plans, special events, and vacations. Many families indicate that, although day care is helpful, occasional total relief from care giving for a more extended period greatly reduces the burden of caring for the person with dementia.

</td></tr>
</table>

Services

Residential Care

The facility was developed to provide a continuum of care to individuals with Alzheimer's disease and dementia at any stage, from the early stages through the end of life.

Day Care

The day care program was developed to benefit participants by providing an environment in which they could achieve and succeed, meet new friends, remain active, and participate in life, as well as to provide support for families. The day care program can accommodate up to five participants at a time and offers full and half-day services. Hours are flexible to meet the needs of participants and families. Participants are encouraged to attend day care at least two days per week initially or more if necessary while becoming adjusted to the program. The day care was slow to develop but now has an average of three to five participants a day.

Day care participants receive meals and snacks and may receive assistance with personal care if individually arranged, in addition to individualized programming and recreational activities. Other services available at the center are negotiated individually, such as beautician services, podiatry, and dentistry.

Respite Care

The respite care program was developed to assist participants and families providing care at home. It has been quite helpful to families in time of crisis and is also utilized as a "test" to determine participants' and families' reaction to the center before long-term placement.

Numerous families make use of respite care several times a year to meet their individual needs for holiday plans, special events, and vacations. Many families indicate that, although day care is helpful, occasional total relief from care giving for a more extended period greatly reduces the burden of caring for the person with dementia.

Education

Part of the mission of the Alois Alzheimer Center is to promote an awareness of the disease and knowledge about progressive programs and creative management techniques. The center established an education component for students to work with staff members who have joint appointments with the center and the University of Cincinnati. The center serves as a clinical setting for students from a variety of disciplines, including nursing, administration, health planning, psychiatry, pharmacy, and gerontology. Initially, student participation was limited by the center to graduate and upper level students prepared to spend long rotations at the center in an effort to moderate the number of unfamiliar others to whom residents would be exposed (a potential source of confusion and anxiety). However, student activity has not been proven to be disruptive to the residents and has, when carefully planned, actually been quite beneficial and enjoyable for students, staff, residents, and families. In particular, staff members derive great satisfaction from contributing to student learning and from being recognized as an educational resource.

The center has collaborated with a variety of individuals, organizations, and facilities locally, nationally, and internationally, sharing information on all aspects of the development of this project and the experience over the past four years. In addition, the center disseminates information through a variety of outreach programs, including a speakers' bureau, educational seminars, presentations, publications, and consultation. Educational programs geared to specific audiences have been developed, including offerings for families, the general community, clergy, nursing assistants, social service personnel, volunteers, activity planners, and other health care professionals.

Research

Planning, coordinating, and conducting research also form an important part of the center's mission. Over the past four years, the center has collaborated with other facilities and various universities—locally and regionally—in many research projects, including an evaluation of a drug utilized to decrease anxiety, the development of an assessment tool to measure subtle cognitive changes in advanced dementia, a formal survey of staff characteristics and satisfaction in specialized facilities, and an examination of the utilization of and satisfaction with respite services.

The entire staff of the center are afforded the opportunity to participate in various research projects. The response has been positive, with most staff and family members wishing to be involved in most projects and frequently suggesting ideas for future research. Administrators note that staff members appreciate the opportunity to contribute to current knowledge and that their involvement in research is related to increased job satisfaction, sense of accomplishment, and self-esteem.

The center does not maintain its own research staff; however, through affiliation with the University of Cincinnati and other regional researchers, the center has established itself as a research-friendly setting with an educated and motivated staff.

All research conducted with center participation takes place on site to facilitate ease of participation for residents and families and to ensure a comfortable and nonthreatening experience for participants. All research results are reported to staff and families in scheduled presentations and during the center's weekly in-service programs held on all three shifts.

Goals
Key therapeutic goals

- *Improve traditional methods of caring* for individuals with AD and other dementias through the development of a physical environment, emotional climate, trained staff, and individualized care plans.
- *Promote the highest level of physical and cognitive functioning possible* for each resident.

- *Minimize the use of restraints*—chemical and physical—through the use of creative behavioral management and an active recreational program.
- *Enrich and enhance the lives of people with dementia* by creating individualized programs that promote accomplishment, self-esteem, a sense of well-being, and joy through a variety of daily activities.
- Establish a philosophy and provide an environment that promote *freedom and choice* within a safe and secure setting.
- Provide mechanisms to *facilitate ongoing family relationships with residents,* such as the development of communication strategies and sponsorship of social events.

Educational goals

- *Establish an initial and ongoing education and support program for staff members* to enhance their ability to provide state-of-the-art care for people with dementia.
- *Provide ongoing education and support programs for families* to decrease stress and promote family involvement.
- *Develop programs to meet the educational needs of the community and the nation* in an attempt to increase awareness of AD while decreasing the myths and fallacies that surround it.
- *Serve as a clinical setting for students* to experience the effects of AD and to observe effective methods of care through clinical rotations.

Research goals

- *Establish the center as a resource to others working in this field* by opening facility doors, sharing experiences, and serving as consultants through presentations and publications, while learning from others.
- *Collaborate locally, nationally, and internationally with researchers* interested in advancing knowledge of AD and dementia and conducting appropriate projects that meet with research board approval.

Political goal

- *Advocate for individuals and families* through routine correspondence with the Ohio Legislature and through promotion of staff involvement in local and national organizations.

Organizational and Social Environment
The staff

Positions and Ratios

The Alois Alzheimer Center is staffed with an executive director, an executive assistant, a director of social service, a director of recreation and activities, activity assistants, a director of nursing, R.N.s, L.P.N.s, a medical records clerk, nursing assistants and orderlies, an office manager and receptionists, and housekeeping, maintenance, laundry, and dietary employees and directors. There are a total of ninety-four full-time and part-time positions at the center.

Organizational Structure and Staffing

Since the facility opened staffing has been adjusted because of a need for more support staff than anticipated in areas such as activities, housekeeping, laundry, and maintenance. An increased number of professional nurses was also necessary (although anticipated), as the residents' acuity level changed over time. Direct care staff to resident ratios, including nursing and activities personnel, are presently 1:5 from 7:00 a.m. to 3:00 p.m., 1:6 from 3:00 p.m. to 11:00 p.m., and 1:10 from 11:00 p.m. to 7:00 a.m.

Training and Hiring

Administrators pay careful attention to the selection of employees to work with cognitively impaired residents at the center. Flexibility, openness, complete understanding of the responsibilities of this type of work, and a high level of individual motivation have been found to be desirable characteristics in prospective employees. Each interview of prospective employees includes a tour of the facility both to increase the interviewee's familiarity with AD and job responsibilities and to observe his or her interactions with residents. Administrators report that this interviewing process has resulted in more appropriate hiring procedures and has subsequently reduced staff turnover, particularly rapid turnover that occurs within a few weeks of hiring.

Once hired, staff members take part in a basic orientation program to orient them to the center and to Alzheimer' disease. New employees participate in a "buddy system" with more experienced personnel in their department to increase familiarity with the environment and the routine and to increase competence in handling difficult situations. Following staff suggestions, a program was implemented in which new employees spend time with two or more persons within their department to expose them to a wide range of experiences and care techniques.

Weekly educational programs offered to staff members on all three shifts are intended to increase staff members' knowledge, sense of support, and contact with each other. Mission clarification is one component of this program to ensure that all employees understand the goals of the facility and share the same vision for resident care. Other programs teach staff members about AD and dementia and give information about management strategies. Various experiences have been incorporated to place staff members in the position of residents and/or family members to increase understanding of the disease and enhance sensitivity. Other topics addressed include sensory changes, loss and grieving, and topics of personal concern to staff members, such as stress identification and reduction. One meeting each month is dedicated to staff discussion with administrators, at which issues addressed include updates and changes and staff members' and administrators' problems and concerns. Policy development and planning also takes place together at these sessions. Reportedly, this participation is related to a greater sense of belonging and ownership in the center.

Morale and Retention

Administrators report that staff morale and retention at the center have been high, although no formal evaluation of turnover has taken place. As the selection and orientation process evolved, administrators noted a tremendous reduction in rapid turnover, particularly of those employees who worked for less than two weeks.

A formal study, "Identification of Staff Characteristics and Job Satisfaction in Working with Individuals with Alzheimer's Disease," conducted at the center included employees from every department. Results indicate that 79 percent found their work satisfying, while 10 percent were unsure and 11 percent did not. Many (83 percent) felt that their work gave them a sense of accomplishment, and most found their work fascinating (64 percent), challenging (79 percent), and not boring (66 percent). Although some felt that their pay was adequate, most believed that they received less than they deserve. Many (67 percent) would probably choose the same occupation again, and even more (77 percent) would advise friends to enter the occupation.

Staff "burnout" is frequently associated with loss and grieving over losses, such as cognitive and functional losses and loss of life. The center offers educational programs on loss and grieving, hosts bereavement specialists to work with staff, and provides memorial services to help staff members deal with these losses.

The residents

Characteristics of the Residents

The Alois Alzheimer Center is a licensed nursing home accommodating eighty-two full-time residents. Designed to provide a continuum of care, the facility receives residents at any stage of the disease. Those entering the center as long-term residents are generally in the moderate to severe stages of dementia. At present, 63 percent of the residents are women and the average age of the residents is seventy-eight years, but residents range in age from fifty-three to ninety-six. Many residents have come to the center from outside the local area, and several came from other states.

Capabilities of residents vary, and no physical impairment excludes them from participating at the center. Residents are assigned to and relocated between the three sections of the facility on the basis of functional and cognitive ability.

Admission and Retention

All individuals participating in programs at the center must have a primary diagnosis of probable Alzheimer's disease or dementia. A secondary diagnosis is considered only if the primary is an acute physical ailment such as a fracture or other temporary condition. Referrals to the center come from a variety of services, doctors, hospital discharge planners, community organizations and agencies, and other families. An interview with a prospective family takes place by phone, where personal information is gathered. If a formal diagnostic assessment has not been completed, it is often recommended and community resources are given. Once the decision has been made to pursue admission, the family is scheduled for a tour of the facility and a meeting with staff members. After this, an assessment of the prospective resident takes place in his or her current living environment by a team from the center, including the director of nursing, the director of social services, and other professionals as required. Evaluative procedures are undertaken before admission to rule out reversible dementias; these procedures include a recent, complete history and physical; the history of medication, alcohol, and caffeine usage; and numerous laboratory assessments.

In addition to medical assessment, staff members gather an extensive personal, social, and dietary history of each resident, which is utilized in the development of an individualized care plan. Staff members also use this information to develop behavioral management strategies and to plan therapeutic activities.

Before the individual becomes a long term resident, a plan is developed to assist with his or her adjustment. Initially, administrators anticipated that adjustment would require several weeks or even months. However, experience demonstrates that residents usually feel quite comfortable within a few weeks, and this has been increasingly true as procedures have been established regarding the admission process. Team assessment also seems to facilitate adjustment, as at least a few staff members are familiar with each new resident. Residents are assigned and located among the three sections of the facility on the basis of functional and cognitive ability, as well as individual social and psychological needs. Families participate in the transition and in all planned activity for the first one or two days as appropriate.

The families

The center's experience has been that, despite the availability of community support programs and services, families demonstrate a great need for support and counseling. Families are encouraged to join or continue participation in community support programs, such as those provided by the Alzheimer's Association. Families vary in the amount of planning of and participation in care that they desire. Staff members work to teach families how to enjoy time with residents in spite of ever-changing communicative losses. Programs and events are designed to allow families to enjoy time with residents without the stress of one-to-one communication.

Families and friends are permitted to visit residents at any time, although the staff must be notified of any visits that must occur between 11:00 p.m. and 7:00 a.m. Monthly meetings for families consist of programs or presentations on various topics, such as information about the disease, care-giving tips, research updates, or information about activities or changes at the center. Refreshments are provided after these presentations, and families often use these opportunities to socialize with staff members and other caregivers.

Program Description

Programs developed at the center focus on individual residents' needs and desires. The goal is to provide as much independence as possible through activities that promote accomplishment and a sense of well-being. Residents are encouraged to do as much as possible for themselves, regardless of extra time demands for staff members.

A large activities staff provides a range of activities geared to individuals at all levels. The activity program is designed to meet the needs of individual residents incapable of filling their own leisure time with meaningful activities. Care is taken to achieve a balance between overstimulation and boredom.

Physical Environment *Description of plan*	The Alois Alzheimer Center is situated on seven acres of land and is surrounded on three sides by a national greenbelt. Because the woods are part of a protected area, no further development may take place on the site, so the quiet, attractive natural setting will be maintained. The site is easily accessible to major thoroughfares.
Principles of spatial arrangement	To accommodate individuals at various levels of cognitive and physical functioning, the facility has naturally evolved into three distinct sections within the single building. Each section has one or more separate activity areas and a dining room.
Entry area	The main entrance to the facility leads to a large lobby area with several large windows and a large skylight, bringing a great deal of natural light indoors. Included is a glass double door, which permits residents to see people coming and going. Administrators report that this is very enjoyable for most residents and that those disturbed by such activity are located away from the lobby.
Outdoor spaces	Locked outdoor courtyards are located outside each exit from the facility. Each is lined with five foot, ivy-covered rod-iron railings designed to create a sense of freedom and nonconfinement. The largest courtyard is open and includes several large, old trees. It includes a grill for cookouts, tables for picnics, gardens, walking areas, and areas for relaxing outdoors under the trees. This courtyard is visible from a variety of locations in the facility. A mulch-covered circular path was developed by volunteers and is used for walks and hikes.
Wandering areas	The facility has wide hallways intended to facilitate wandering. Double security-coded doors within the hallways divide the facility and can be used to restrict access to particular areas. Auditory and visual door alarms are linked to a central monitoring station, enabling staff members to be aware of residents leaving the facility. All individuals have physical access to the entire facility, although most residents spend the majority of their time in their own areas. Administrators feel that wandering subsides with the freedom to wander if desired.
Living rooms and social spaces	The noninstitutional interior design is intended to be uncluttered and attractive, in the style of traditional living rooms. There are several large and small living room areas decorated in soft colors. Floors are carpeted in the hallways and in many residents' rooms. Several small alcoves have been furnished as living areas and gathering places. A large living room is separated from the dining area by a half wall; it includes a functional fireplace, a piano, and a stereo system. This room often serves as the site for musical programs. The large number of social spaces easily accommodates isolation of agitated residents.
Kitchen/dining areas	The three separate dining rooms are designed to address the needs of the specific resident populations dining there. Each room was modified to limit stim-

ulation and encourage eating. The main dining area has two seatings to reduce the number of residents eating at one time and to accommodate differences in capabilities. The first seating includes those individuals capable of managing more stimulation in their environment while maintaining the ability to concentrate on their meals. This group enjoys music during meals; the piano is frequently played during lunch hour. The residents seem to enjoy this, often stopping and clapping after a song. The second seating includes residents who require lower levels of stimulation and can tolerate little distraction. No music is played during this seating.

Cooking and food preparation activities often take place in the large dining room, although there is no kitchen to which residents have access. The large dining/living room in the central area of the complex is used to accommodate large groups for family activities and entertainment.

Residents' rooms

Residents' rooms range in size from 300 to 400 square feet, each with a separate, closed bathroom and shower. Residents are permitted to bring furniture from home to personalize their rooms. Because of the facility's previous function, all resident rooms and community areas have very large windows that allow abundant natural light into the facility. Private rooms are assigned to individuals who, because of manageability or compatibility, require a private room. One of the largest rooms can accommodate three residents, and assignment depends upon individual needs and compatibility. Administrators report that most individuals function well in semiprivate rooms. Many friendships are attributed to the fact that residents share rooms, and staff members report that tasks accomplished by roommates might not be accomplished by residents independently.

Residents' rooms are identified by name plates, a meaningful fixture on the door such as a hat or photo, and personalized interior decoration. The experience of staff members has been that residents can find their own rooms without assistance to a certain point in the disease process and that, beyond that, little can be done except for direct guidance.

Toilet and shower/ tub rooms

Each resident room has a personal bathroom with a toilet and shower. Administrators believe that individual bathrooms with showers facilitate personal care for many residents. In addition, there is a central bathing area with a large shower and whirlpool tub.

Equipment and furnishings

Walls are used for most decorating, as residents tend to carry off items left on tables and hutches.

Materials and surfaces

Initially, the entire facility was carpeted, but some areas have been converted to vinyl because of high maintenance requirements.

Alzheimer's Care Center

Address	154 Dresden Avenue Gardiner, ME 04345 (207) 626-1771
Owner	Kennebec Long-Term Care of Kennebec Health Systems
Staff contact	Jessie E. Jacques, R.N., Administrator
Facility type	Boarding home with respite and day care
License	Nonprofit; boarding home facility
Residents	28 boarding home residents, 2 respite residents, and 6–10 day care clients
Staff	2 L.P.N.s, 1½ housekeepers, an administrator, an activities director, a social worker, a receptionist, a dietary aide, and 26 resident aides
Staff to resident ratio	1:5 from 7:00 a.m. to 11:00 p.m.; 1:10 from 11:00 p.m. to 7:00 a.m.
Site/context	Located in a residential section of a small town, adjacent to a medical complex and a natural wooded area
Size	11,500 square feet (approximate)
Date of completion	1988
Architect	Paul Stevens, of Stevens, Morton, Rose & Thompson

Figure 2.2   Plan of the Alzheimer's Care Center, Gardiner, Maine.

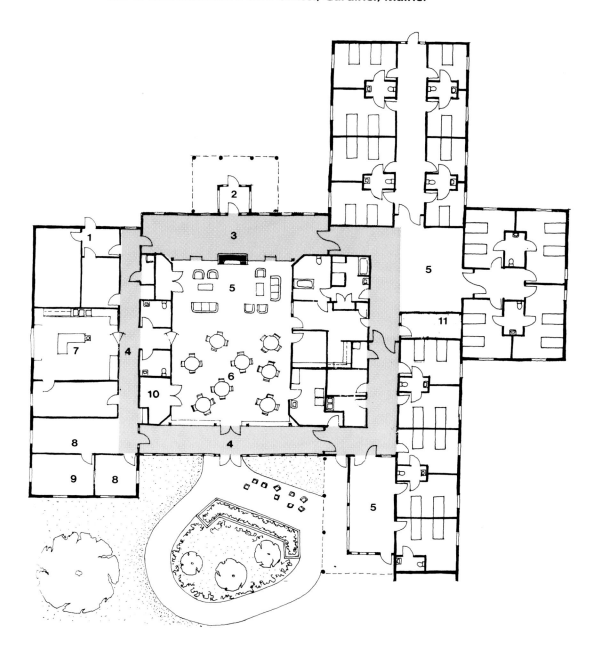

1 new entrance	**5** living rooms	**8** administration
2 original entrance	**6** dining room/activity area	**9** conference room
3 original lobby		**10** serving kitchen
4 wandering path	**7** kitchen	**11** grooming area

Residential Clusters

+ Residents' rooms are clustered in three groups; access to each cluster is free but can be controlled by a lockable door. Each cluster is associated with a small living room.

Wandering Path

− A good portion of the internal wandering path is an ordinary corridor; the better section overlooks the outdoor courtyard and the great room. The circulation is continuous but may be interrupted if one of the units requires isolation.

Positive Outdoor Space

+ The secure outdoor courtyard is furnished with seating, a planter, and a paved, continuous path. The yard is adjacent to the living room porch and provides degrees of shelter and a positive microclimate.

Activity Alcoves

+ The house includes several varied activity spaces.

+ The great room's working fireplace and warm decor contribute to a domestic feeling.

+ The kitchen serves as a focal point for numerous food-related activities with residents.

− The large size of the great room detracts from the residential nature of this space.

Noninstitutional Environment

+ The building's form and construction, the outdoor courtyard, and most residents' rooms radiate a domestic and residential image.

− The kitchen is a large, institutional food-processing facility, with no physical connection to residents' activity spaces.

Entry and Transition Space

− The original main entry (2) was located on the main wandering path, where it overlooked the great room. The direct exposure to frequent "coming and going" caused much disruption and agitation, and the entry was later moved to a more discreet location (1).

Background

History

The Alzheimer Care Center in Gardiner, Maine, is a nonprofit, boarding home and day care/respite facility developed specifically to meet the needs of people with dementia. The facility was devised as a home for people in the early stages of the disease who do not yet need the round-the-clock medical care a nursing home provides. When opened, the center was the only boarding facility in the country designed exclusively for the care of people in the early and middle stages of Alzheimer's disease. It is owned by Kennebec Long-Term Care Corporation, a division of Kennebec Health System. The Alzheimer Care Center is situated next to the Gardiner Division of Kennebec Valley Medical Center, a twenty-nine-bed skilled nursing facility with X-ray and laboratory services, as well as outpatient eye surgery facilities. The medical center is also a division of Kennebec Health System.

Mission

The Alzheimer Care Center was developed as a joint public/private experiment to examine new methods of caring for the state's population with Alzheimer's disease. A multidisciplinary planning committee composed of consumers, medical and mental health care providers, representatives of state and federal governments, and facility designers convened in 1984 to study the needs of Maine's people with AD, as outlined by the Task Force on Mental Health Services to Elderly Persons. The task force had suggested a review of boarding home regulations to serve AD clients better and had recommended that a broad education and training program be developed to upgrade formal care-giving skills throughout the state.

Funding

The state's experiment was intended to suggest models for AD resource allocation and education for other states. Its financial structure and development process also serve as a model for other innovative facilities. To finance planning and implementation of the facility, the Bureau of Maine's Elderly developed a grant proposal and submitted it to the federal Administration on Aging. Upon approval, a two-year, $275,000 grant was awarded to develop the project.

The financial risks of start-up for the $1 million center were shared by the public and private sectors, with the latter assuming responsibility for all construction costs. Yankee Healthcare was successful in securing permanent financing through a loan under the Essential Community Facilities Program of the Farmer's Home Administration. Before the granting of this loan, the staff of the Farmer's Home Administration had never reviewed an application for a boarding care facility strictly serving the needs of Alzheimer's patients. The decision may signal a breakthrough in opportunity for facility planners everywhere.

Current costs

Ongoing financing and management of the Alzheimer's Care Center is provided by Kennebec Long-Term Care, a private, nonprofit corporation. Also crucial to the operation of the facility are funds that its residents receive under a state assistance program for financially eligible persons, together with special allowances for intensive staffing requirements to service populations with special needs. The current actual cost of providing boarding care is $80 per day for the thirty beds (full time and respite). Maine's Bureau of Medical Services made available $65 a day to support state-assisted residents of the facility ($15 less than the cost of care). Because the boarding home is not a "medical" facility, these funds are not Medicaid. They come, instead, from the state's Supplemental Security Income Fund, which pays for residential care. Since March 1991, Medicaid has also become involved in the funding.

Self-pay residents pay $92 a day, which is intended to cover both the cost of providing care to those residents as well as the payment shortfall for state-assisted residents, compared to charges of about $80 to $115 a day at a central Maine nursing home. The $65 a day contributed by the state represents a "special circumstance" payment rate that was negotiated for the boarding care facility; the rate established recognizes the necessity for an increased level of staffing for the care of people with Alzheimer's disease. About 45–50 percent of boarding residents are covered by state funds. Respite care residents pay $97 per day. The center also provides approximately four hundred hours of day care per month, for which state and self-pay clients pay $6.75 per hour.

Fuel and insurance, workers' compensation, and employee insurance costs have all risen significantly since the opening of the facility, causing some reorganization of the center's finances. Although the Alzheimer Care Center lost $32,641 in its first full year of operation, results for the first three months of fiscal year 1992 indicate that a modest excess of revenue over expenses will be achieved in the current year. Improved financial performance is attributable to negotiated increases in state reimbursement levels, higher respite care occupancy, and increased utilization of the day care facility.

Proponents of the center emphasize that, while costs may be only marginally less than nursing home placement, residents' quality of life and family satisfaction may be higher and resistance to placement lower. (The latter of these may not necessarily be a desirable outcome, given recent attention to the benefits associated with continued residence in the community.)

Services

The original grant called for the establishment of a continuum of services and programs by combining four components, collectively titled the Alzheimer's Project of Kennebec Valley: (1) the Alzheimer Care Center boarding home, (2) a geriatric evaluation unit (GEU) to assess individuals possibly afflicted with Alzheimer's disease, (3) a day care and respite program, and (4) a community resource center to provide information and training for both professional and family caregivers.

The Boarding Home

The boarding home portion of the Alzheimer Care Center opened in February 1988, with all twenty-eight resident positions occupied. Residents were admitted gradually over the first three-month period, at the rate of about two to four per week. The center has served as the home for both the boarding center and the day and respite service, which are fully integrated. The Community Resource Center is also located within this facility.

The Geriatric Evaluation Unit

The GEU is headquartered in the building adjacent to the Alzheimer Care Center. The GEU has evaluated over seven hundred individuals in the past six years and has generated a waiting list of names. The team serves as the regional resource for systematic evaluations of persons suffering from dementias.

Day and Respite Care

The day care program began in July 1988. The program experienced a temporary initial slump in membership as many of the day care participants became full-time residents of the facility. This trend had both positive and negative implications, as it eased transition for residents, family, and staff, yet depleted the day care population as a source of financial revenue for the facility in the interim. More consistent recruitment of day care participants has resolved this problem, and the day care population has stabilized at approximately ten members.

The day care program offers both half- and full-time schedules and is very flexible in the hours its members may attend. Staff members encourage participants to attend at least two days a week to assure adjustment to the program. The program includes meals and a snack, personal care, use of the whirlpool, exercise and activities, and the services of a beautician. Day care is provided weekdays from 7:00 a.m. to 5:00 p.m.; extension of this service to weekends is also being considered.

The respite program officially began in June 1988, after the residential portion of the project was fully implemented. Only one of the two respite beds was fully utilized during the first year. Informal marketing and contacting of families on the waiting list have led to full occupancy since May 1989. Respite care is available in durations ranging from one to six weeks, with the average visit lasting two weeks. Two beds are provided for respite on a continuing basis. The goal of the program is to ensure that respite is available in a predictable, scheduled way, not just when caregivers "can't take it any more." The two beds are currently reserved four to five months in advance. In a survey of their satisfaction with the facility and its services, many families indicated that the respite service was very useful and that they would use it more often if financial assistance were available. The beds have been used by families considering placement in the home, and the experience has helped family members work through the placement decision and allowed the staff to assess the appropriateness of the individual to the facility and vice versa. Administrators strongly recommend that similar facilities include respite among their services.

The Community Resource Center

The Community Resource Center contains mechanisms for disseminating information statewide. A variety of training, outreach, and technical assistance efforts have been made by the center, including publication of the results of start-up and operational experiences with the boarding home. In addition, the resource center sponsors two support groups for family members and offers two-hour orientation classes and a tour of the center every eight weeks. The center regularly hosts student interns throughout the academic year.

Research

Research is an important component of the center, although this facet has not been as well developed as other components of the project. The Alzheimer Care Center is supported in this aim by cooperation with the director of research of Kennebec Long-Term Care, who helps to propose, coordinate, direct, and evaluate research in and of the facility. Research efforts to date include a nursing home linkage study to determine the potential relationship between regional nursing homes and the project before its opening, a formal survey of family members' satisfaction with the project, and a special research project assessing the effects on residents of efforts to reduce noise levels in the facility.

Current status

After three years of operation, the Alzheimer Care Center is considered a success by its developers and administrators, primarily because of the special design of the building, the well-chosen, well-trained staff, and the excellent activity program (the second two of which are also aided by the design). The boarding home, day care, and respite services are all filled to capacity. The facility now receives almost daily inquiries from architects, developers, and professional caregivers from around the country.

Goals of the Facility

The ultimate purpose of the Alzheimer Care Center is better understanding of people in the first and second stages of the disease. The major emphasis of the center is on quality of life for residents and their families, supported by a non-medical, noninstitutional environment and program. The facility attempts to offer a sense of structure with flexibility; activities are of utmost importance in this regard.

Key therapeutic goals

- *Improve residents' quality of life* through appropriate activities and a supportive environment.
- *Maximize abilities* by providing a range of experiences for residents of different functional and cognitive levels.

Organizational and Social Environment
The staff

Positions and Ratios

The Alzheimer Care Center is staffed with an administrator, social worker, licensed practical nurse, full-time activities director, separate day care coordinator, and several aides each shift. A total of thirty-one employees provide direct care to residents.

Organizational Structure and Staffing: Adjusting to Higher Levels

After the opening of the facility, it became immediately obvious that intended staffing levels for the facility were insufficient. New residents required more time and more one-on-one attention while adjusting to the facility than had been anticipated. Staff members have determined that residents require approximately two months to adjust to life in the center. The adjusted typical staffing pattern includes one L.P.N. and four resident aides from 7:00 a.m. to 3:00 p.m., the same from 3:00 p.m. to 11:00 p.m., and three aides from 11:00 p.m. to 7:00 a.m.

Hiring and Training: Nontraditional Backgrounds Preferred

The staff of the Alzheimer's Care Center was hired in January 1988, at which time a two-week training session was completed by all employees. Efforts were made to seek staff members with other than traditional nursing, nursing home, or long-term care backgrounds, as these individuals might demonstrate preconceived biases regarding people with dementia. Emphasis is placed on teaching staff members to regard residents as individuals and to help residents to regain self-esteem.

In the first week of training, the GEU team described the diagnostic process, national and local speakers and films were used to describe the process of caring for people with dementia, and team-building sessions were held. This training period provided the opportunity for staff to become acquainted with each other and with the philosophy of the home. During the second week, orientation and preparation for intake activities included visits to AD units of intermediate care (nursing home) facilities. Staff members from all shifts also met as a group with family members to discuss their concerns and to identify the special characteristics and needs of each resident.

Morale and Retention: Methods for Keeping Both High

Staff morale has remained high in the center. The center replaces approximately 1.5 employees yearly. Reasons for the center's high employee retention rate may include the following factors.

1. The staff to resident ratio on some shifts is as high as 1:5.

2. The facility very carefully selected employees who want to work with people with dementia in this type of environment. Most of the staff hired as resident aides had no previous nursing or nursing home experience or training; thus, there was no need to unlearn work habits more appropriate to other settings (e.g., strict schedule of bed changing, cleaning, toileting). Similarly, for most of the staff, negative attitudes and stereotypes about AD based on experiences caring for residents in the late stages of the disease did not need to be addressed.

3. There is an emphasis on ongoing staff development and education. Periodic in-service training is provided, and tuition assistance is available for those who want to pursue additional certification.

4. Opportunities are provided for staff to share ideas and concerns at regular staff meetings.

The residents

Characteristics of the Residents

The Alzheimer Care Center is designed to provide for twenty-eight boarding home residents, two respite clients, and ten day care participants. It is currently at full capacity. The sex distribution of residents is currently twenty-six women and two men, with more men than women in the day care program. The average age is seventy-five, and residents are sixty-six to ninety years old. Approximately 50 percent of the residents come to the facility from outside the local area.

All residents are ambulatory and able to do at least some self-care with help upon admission to the center. An evaluation of activities of daily living of residents identified 20 percent capable of total self-care, 7 percent needing minimal care, 33 percent needing moderate care, and 40 percent needing total care.

Many of the residents became incontinent to varying degrees after entering the home. Staff and administrators have concluded that, in this setting, mild incontinence (occasional inappropriate voiding) should not be the sole reason for discharging a resident. In addition, the GEU team has become more specific in its questions regarding incontinence to identify those residents who may have more serious forms of incontinence.

Admission and Retention: Refining Boarding Home Criteria

An assessment by the Geriatric Evaluation Unit is necessary for acceptance into the residential and respite programs and is strongly encouraged for those entering the day care program. State of Maine boarding home criteria were used for selection (ambulatory, continent, self-feeding). In addition, to avoid short-term placements, the center evaluated past medical history to determine the likelihood of the individual maintaining these skills and overall health for at least one year. Of the original residents, twenty (71 percent) came to the facility from their own or their children's homes, one (4 percent) from a boarding home, and seven (25 percent) from intermediate care (nursing home) facilities. Of the seven residents who came from intermediate care facilities, all improved in overall functioning after placement at the facility and four have remained in the facility and are doing well. Many of the current residents now come to the program after participation in the day care and respite programs.

A fourteen-item discharge scoring guideline developed for the boarding home examines residents' responses to specific criteria in the subareas of incontinence, activities of daily living, feeding, and mobility. Residents who score less than a predetermined number of the twenty possible points on the guideline are usually recommended for discharge, although staff members also evaluate the level to which residents continue to benefit from the center's environment and programs and make efforts to retain residents who continue to benefit greatly from the center.

During the center's first two years of operation, twenty people were discharged: four to hospitals for medical reasons, fifteen to intermediate care facilities because of deterioration in mental and physical functioning, and one to the state mental hospital. The staff continue to document the reasons for discharge to develop a profile of persons most likely to remain at the home for an extended period of time.

The families

Families are encouraged to participate at the home. A recent survey of family members indicated a very high level of satisfaction with the home. Because family members are encouraged to participate in the initial evaluation sessions (GEU), staff believe that families have more information and are better able to cope with placement. Despite efforts to organize activities to involve families, administrators have found that many family members gradually reduce contact with residents after they become comfortable with and confident of the care provided at the home.

Description of the Program

Activities are the great thrust and primary emphasis of the Alzheimer Care Center, evidenced by the employment of a full-time activities director. All residents (boarding home, respite, and day care) are integrated into the same activity spaces and programs. These activities include music, exercise, discussion groups, field trips, entertainment, pet therapy, and child therapy. Resident aides and volunteers are oriented to the importance of activities for helping residents to develop and maintain a meaningful quality of life.

The daily activities offer a structured, consistent routine, as well as opportunities for social interaction. Mornings begin with the daily discussion group, with topics ranging from local history to current events or upcoming holidays. Music is important—one resident plays the piano, accompanying the group in frequent sing-a-longs; a second resident used to play guitar and now plays harmonica, and visiting musical groups perform at the facility at least twice monthly. Field trips outside the center are also frequent for high-functioning residents. Nearly 50 percent of the residents can be taken out for at least some types of activities (although lack of transportation limits the number of residents that can leave the facility at any one time). In the past, residents have gone maple sugaring and apple picking, to country fairs, and on a visit to Swan's Island. Efforts are made to avoid activities that are overstimulating for residents, as this has been an occasional problem.

Household-based activities are also central to the activities program and include jobs such as linen folding, dusting, clearing tables, setting table, food preparation, and sorting projects. Social events may consist of teas, coffee hours, ice cream parties, picnics, and local entertainment. Residents regularly take part in a variety of exercises conducted by the activities director and resident aides, such as table ball, "gerobics," chair exercises, and play with a colorful parachute. Pets have been successfully introduced into the facility and currently include three cats and a parakeet. A former seeing eye dog also resided in the facility at one time. The administrator's dog now visits occasionally. This portion of the project is under the direction of a local veterinarian.

Structured group activities are planned on at least an hourly basis throughout the day, with fewer activities planned for weekends. Activities are always scheduled during the staggered shift changes, as this is a time when residents frequently become agitated or confused. All activities are geared to individual interest, abilities, and self-fulfillment/satisfaction requirements. The building design allows parallel (simultaneous) programming of as many as three small and/or large group activities. Staff members also tend to the needs of those individuals not involved in group activities. Efforts are made to plan activities for both high- and low-functioning residents. In addition, the staff carefully observe the scheduled quiet periods to allow residents to rest and relax.

Visiting

The center maintains an open policy regarding visiting. Family members and friends are also encouraged to take residents out of the facility for day trips and longer visits. The center plans regular activities to encourage visiting and participation, such as barbecues and other social events. Family members of day care participants are much more likely than those of boarding home residents to attend these events, perhaps because of the process of withdrawal following placement (described earlier). Family members are more likely to visit at their own convenience, and almost all caregivers faithfully attend the quarterly team conferences, during which the status of each resident is reviewed with his or her family members.

Physical Environment
The context

The Alzheimer Care Center is located in a quiet wooded area near a residential section of stately homes in the small town of Gardiner in central Maine, just outside of the capital city of Augusta. The center sits at the bottom of a hill, below the Kennebec Valley Medical Center's Gardiner Division.

The role of the environment

The facility strives for a tranquil atmosphere inside and out. A calm, non-threatening environment and appropriate communication strategies are used to address most behavioral problems. Monitoring and adjusting the environment is an ongoing process at the center.

Entry area

Traditional in style, the single-story clapboard building has a front, spacious, central entrance that is no longer in use and a second front service door, now used as the primary entrance. The original main entrance in the front lobby had been fitted with a sophisticated alarm system to control wandering; however, it was very visible to residents from the great room. Constant entering and departing of staff members, caregivers, visitors, and others had been disconcerting and disturbing to residents. Consequently, the out-of-the-way service entrance was adopted as the "main" entrance, causing a significant drop in agitation associated with entering and departing. This entrance is accessible via two separate interior doors, useful when a resident has followed a person who is leaving and is standing at the door when another person arrives.

Great room

Inside the center, the great room is comfortable and homey, decorated in bright colors. Winslow Homer prints hang on the walls. Large windows in the surrounding wandering path let in plenty of light. In the living room portion of the great room, a fireplace is surrounded by overstuffed easy chairs and sofas. Carpeting covers the floor. There is a piano along one wall, a centerpiece of the activity program. One resident, a former commercial artist, and her daughter helped with the interior design, selecting some of the pictures for the walls and suggesting hues for color coding aimed at helping people with dementia find their way.

The second half of the great room is used as the dining and activity area. It is furnished with colonial maple chairs and tables for four residents, to accommodate family-style dining. Tile floors were chosen for easy cleanup after meals and activities. Wallpaper with fruits and vegetables is used as a visual cue for residents to remind them of the function of this space.

Despite the spatial division and domestic decor, the large size of the great room is rather institutional.

Wandering path

The open layout encourages wandering in the carpeted hallways that loop throughout the facility. A circular path is formed around the great room, administrative hall and kitchen, and bedroom corridor.

Activity spaces

In addition to the great room, two other activity spaces can accommodate simultaneous programmed and unprogrammed activities of large or small groups of residents. The first of these is the bright, floral living room associated with two resident rooms on the southern wing of the building. This space includes a row of easy chairs and abundant sunlight from the abutting backyard. This is a quiet area that is typically used for the isolation of agitated residents and quiet activities.

A second "living room" is located between two additional wings of resident rooms. A semicircle of easy chairs and sofas surrounds the television set— viewed very selectively, according to staff members. This space is livelier than the first living room, situated as it is along the wandering path, between two wings of bedrooms, and near to the staff lounge and nurses' station.

The services of a fully functional beauty shop are available for the use of both boarding home and day care participants.

A small smoking room also serves as an activity space of sorts. This space resembles a typical employee break room; all smoking materials are kept in this locked room.

Kitchen

All meals for the residents are brought to the center by golf cart from the medical facility kitchen at the top of the hill. A spacious kitchen is used primarily by residents for food preparation activities, such as making sandwiches and salads and frosting cookies for weekly picnics. The kitchen contains sufficient counter space for many residents to work at once; however, it is somewhat stark and institutional in appearance. The kitchen is located across the hall from a serving kitchen that connects directly to the dining room.

Residents' rooms

Wooden doors with a punch-code security system separate the residential wings from the great room; although these are normally kept open, they can be shut to isolate an agitated resident from the rest of the group, if necessary. Residence wings are distinguished by different colors and wallpaper motifs to create individualized living areas and to aid residents in locating their rooms. The center has thirteen semiprivate and four private rooms, with two private rooms reserved for in-house respite. There is no difference in cost to residents for a private versus a shared room.

Figure 2.3

Personalization of residents rooms enhances the noninstitutional image of the facility and may help residents to identify their own spaces. (Courtesy of Alzheimer Care Center; Gardiner, Maine.)

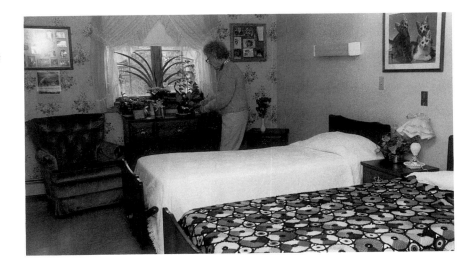

Each room is identified with a name plate and a framed photograph of the resident, many from the past. Residents are encouraged to bring prints, photos, and other personal items from home to decorate and personalize their rooms (fig. 2.3). Old-fashioned wallpaper patterns, chosen to be familiar and attractive to the residents, were selected for each room. Each resident has a twin bed, a dresser, and a chair provided by the center, and all resident rooms are equipped with built-in closets.

Staff members feel that the small size of residents' rooms can be viewed as a positive feature, as this forces socializing to occur outside of bedrooms. Staff members have also found that private rooms and baths are much more functional than shared facilities, particularly for the management of toileting.

Toilet and shower/ tub rooms

The boarding home has one shower, one conventional tub, and one Century whirlpool with a hydraulic lift. The conventional tub is rarely used. One or two of the residents occasionally use the shower, but most use the whirlpool tub with the hydraulic lift on a regular basis. Administrators suggest that, for this generation, bathing in a tub is more familiar than showering, except possibly for some male residents who may be familiar with showers from participating in sports throughout their lives.

Most residents share a toilet room between two shared bedrooms. Incontinence has proven to be a bigger problem in the facility than was originally anticipated. Many residents became incontinent upon entering the center; for others, the actual degree of their incontinence was not detected in the original GEU. Strategies to deal with this are administrative, programmatic, and environmental. Administrative strategies include more detailed questions regarding incontinence in the original GEU, as well as the decision that mild and occasional bladder incontinence should not constitute a reason for dismissal from the center. Programmatic strategies include bowel/bladder work-ups and regular two hour toileting; housekeeping is also considered part of the care plan. Finally, environmental strategies include painting toilet seats a bright color to help residents identify the toilet and the application of soil-resistant materials throughout the facility to accommodate the occasionally incontinent resident.

All residents' toiletry articles are kept in a central, locked closet in labeled bins, to prevent rummaging.

Administrative and staff areas

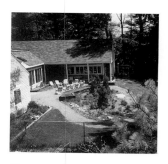

Figure 2.4
Overview of the outdoor space, seating area, and wandering path. The non-institutional building partially defines the backyard on three sides.

The service wing of the facility includes an open reception area, the private office of the administrator, and a small conference room. Both the reception area and the administrative office are open to wandering residents when occupied. Staff members have found that residents who spend a great deal of time in the quiet administrative area are frequently those residents who can no longer tolerate the noise or stimulation of group activities or other residents and who are frequently soon dismissed from the center (although residents also vary individually in the amount of stimulation they can tolerate or enjoy).

The small conference room is occasionally rented out to local groups for meetings, which brings in additional revenue and, more importantly, destigmatizes the facility and its residents while increasing the pool of local citizens who are familiar with the facility's goals and needs.

The nurses' station is located in a central core of staff spaces, and the bathing rooms are in a space that was formerly used exclusively as a staff lounge. The station was too accessible to residents in its prior location in the middle of this hall, causing a great deal of resident traffic and rummaging in staff papers. A locked examination and medicine storage room is located adjacent to the nurses' room.

Outdoor spaces

The building is surrounded by a natural, wooded area; residents often accompany the activity director on walks in the nearby woods as a part of the programmed activity schedule. The doors to the backyard are normally kept open in nice weather. A second outside door from the residential wing (not visible from the great room) is controlled by a punch-code security system. Behind the center is a paved patio equipped with lawn furniture, overlooking a large flower and vegetable garden (fig. 2.4). The garden is tended by residents, with assistance from staff members. This outdoor area is a popular destination for visiting.

Equipment and furnishings

Efforts are made to introduce noninstitutional furnishings throughout the facility, particularly in the great room, living rooms, and resident rooms. With the exception of framed prints in one living room and corridor, no loose materials—such as wall hangings or decorations—are permitted because these serve as temptations to tampering by residents.

Materials and surfaces

In general, hardware and materials and surfaces have undergone extensive wear since their installation. Administrators particularly recommend high-quality, strong, durable, and incontinence-proof materials and hardware.

Alzheimer's Disease Residential Center, California Pacific Medical Center

Address	225 30th Street San Francisco, CA 94131 (415) 550-2200
Owner	Senior Services Division, California Pacific Medical Center
Staff contact	Janeane Randolph, Director
Facility type	Long-term care facility, with one respite bed
Residents	20 long-term care residents and 1 respite client
Staff	Five day-shift, direct care employees; two night-shift, direct care employees. Staff will include an R.N. director, a recreational therapist, a social worker, resident assistants, and L.P.N.s. Clerical support will be provided by the central office of the Senior Services Division.
Staff to resident ratio	1:4 for the day shift; 1:8 or 1:10 for the evening shift
Site/context	One floor of a three-story medical facility located in a residential neighborhood in San Francisco
Size	9,500 square feet (approximate)
Date of completion	(Expected) 1994
Architects	Original and final design: Barker Associates, Palo Alto, Calif.
Schematic proposals for revisions	Uriel Cohen and Gerald Weisman, Milwaukee, Wis.

This case study is presented as an illustration of a number of possible alternative applications of important design principles in the context of a major renovation project. Each alternative highlights several different design approaches aimed at resolving the same primary goals. The client and architect used the proposed revisions as design guidance for the development of the final design.

Figure 2.5   Plans for the Alzheimer's Disease Residential Center, San Francisco, California.
Existing floor plan of the setting for the proposed unit.

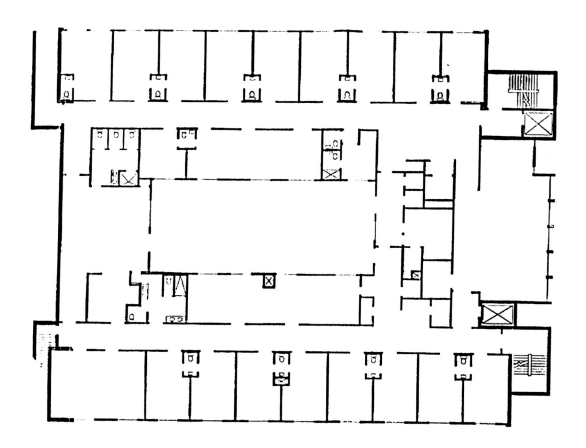

First schematic design proposal for renovation.

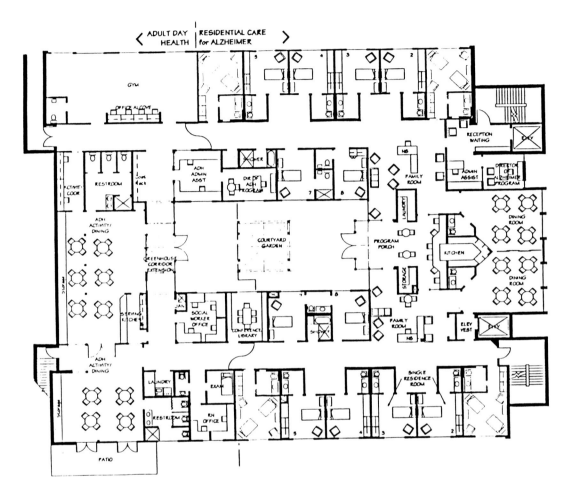

(Drawing by Barker Associates, Architects.)

Figure 2.6   Revision 1: Plan. Design and drawing by Cohen/Weisman.

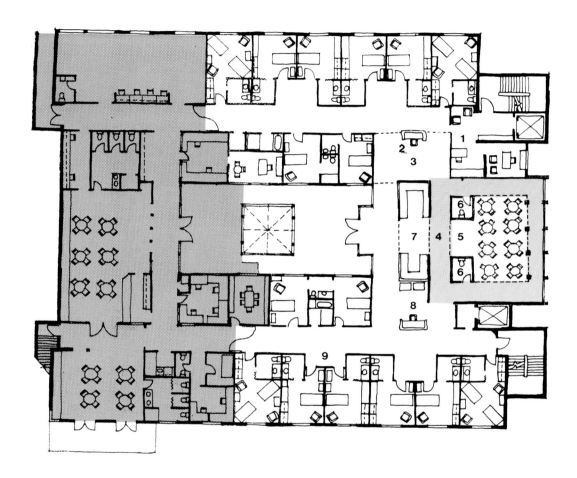

1   entry

2   control point; work space for a staff member provides an unobtrusive surveillance point.

3   family room or activity space

4   wandering path around dining/ activity space

5   dining area may be partitioned into two intimate areas. These can double as activity areas.

6   toilet rooms—accessible but discreet

7   serving kitchen; this can become a locus for other activities, such as washing and drying dishes or folding linen.

8   work space for staff members is associated with activity space.

9   smaller area for an entry zone to each bedroom; added storage is provided in the room. This could include a personal display box.

Figure 2.7   Revision 2: Plan. Design and drawing by Cohen/Weisman.

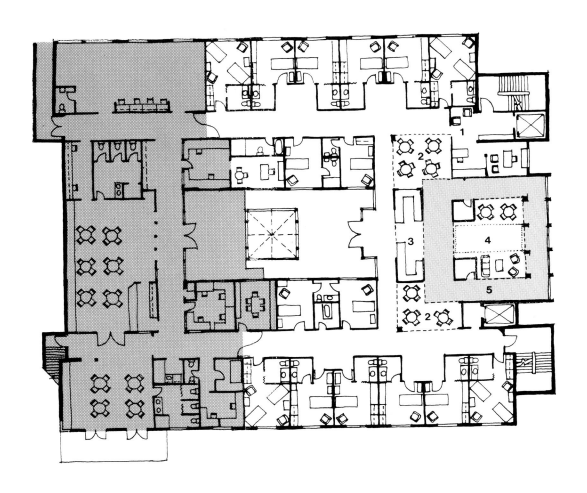

1   entry

2   intimate dining; two separate areas are linked to two respective residential clusters.

3   central "domestic" kitchen; it is located for unobtrusive surveillance to most public areas.

4   living/family rooms; these are potential spaces for other activities.

5   wandering path overlooks activities and dining areas.

Figure 2.8   **Revision 3: Plan. Design and drawing by Cohen/Weisman.**

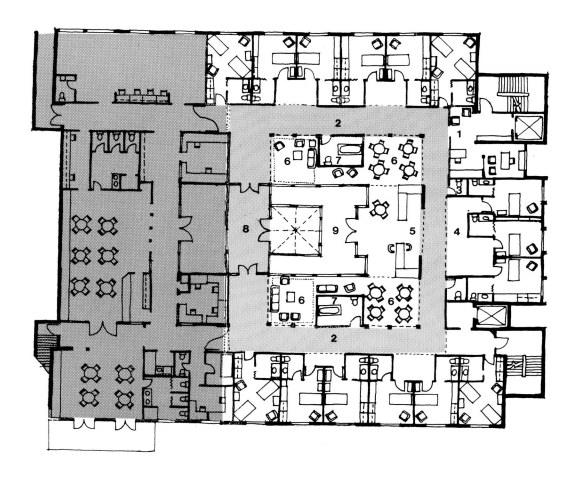

1   entry

2   wandering path overlooking activity
    spaces

3   toilet room, accessible to public
    areas

4   small cluster of residents' rooms

5   serving kitchen, an unobtrusive ob-
    servation point, overlooking most
    public areas, entries to residents'
    rooms, and outdoor space

6   various activity areas: living room,
    intimate dining area, and sitting
    area. Each public zone is associated
    with a respective residential cluster

7   assisted bathing area

8   optional greenhouse passage. If the
    optional passage is not imple-
    mented, this section can be added
    to activity areas

9   outdoor court and garden

Figure 2.9   Plan. Final solution by the architect and client, integrating and incorporating many design features and concepts proposed in the previous three revisions. (Drawing by Barker Associates, Architects.)

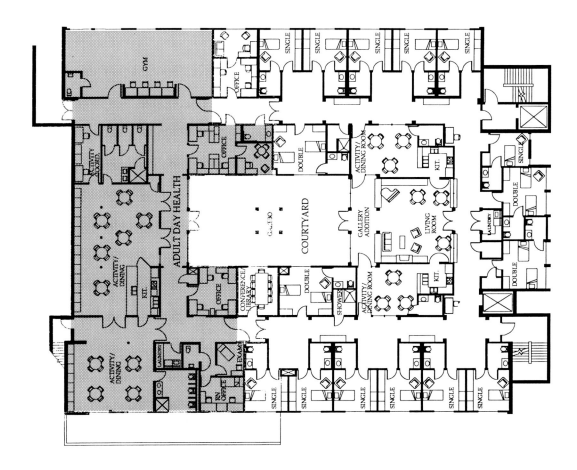

Background

History

Senior Services of California Pacific Medical Center (formerly Pacific Presbyterian Medical Center and Children's Hospital) established a large, multipurpose senior center in 1979. The commitment to develop a unique, non-nursing home residential program for people with Alzheimer's disease and related dementias was approved by the board in 1990. A capital campaign to raise over two million dollars is nearly finalized, and construction of the first phase of the project is due to begin in 1992.

Since 1980, services and programs have been added to form San Francisco's most comprehensive continuum of elder care. Services provided by the center include several senior dining rooms located throughout the city, a home-delivered meal program, the Adult Day Health Care Center, San Francisco's first Alzheimer's Day Care Resource Center, the Retired Senior Volunteer Program, "VIP"—a model service exchange program, case management, transportation, and other services.

Mission

The Alzheimer's Disease Residential Center will provide care to people with dementia, as well as serve as a model site for training. It will include a strong focus on research into the provision of a high-quality life to severely confused individuals.

Costs

There is currently no third-party reimbursement for this type of care in California. The charge for care is projected at approximately $95.00 a day for private-pay clients. For those unable to afford this charge, limited endowment funds will be available to provide care on a sliding fee scale.

Services

The residential program will offer twenty long-term care beds and one respite care bed. Specialized services and features will include medical and dental care, social work services, family counseling, caregiver support groups, a lending resource library, a beauty shop, and a specialized acute care geropsychiatric program available through the main hospital.

Adjacent to the residential unit are facilities for adult day health care and Alzheimer's day care for people with dementia, with openings for sixty participants per day.

Goals

Therapeutic and family-oriented goals

- *Provide resident care that residents and families experience as safe, enjoyable, and enriching* and that enables residents to live life as fully as their disease permits.
- *Establish a relationship with families that is supportive* and that facilitates a partnership in care.

Educational and research-oriented goals

- Share expertise in resident care through educational programs offered to the greater community and by serving as a statewide and national demonstration site.
- *Conduct research that advances the knowledge of appropriate care.*
- *Support replication of the program and collaboration in research internationally.*

Programs	The focus of the program will be on activities that engage residents, are failure-free, and support remaining abilities and functions. The program emphasizes opportunities to move through spaces that engage attention and provide opportunities for exercise and participation in activities of normal daily life.
The Staff *Positions and ratios*	The staff will include an R.N. director, a recreational therapist, a social worker, resident assistants, and L.P.N.s. Clerical support will be provided by the central office of Senior Services.
Staffing ratios	Estimated staff to resident ratios will be 1:5 during the day and evening shifts and 1:7 at night.
Training	Staff will be given advance training as well as continuing in-service training. The center will also serve as a training site for professionals in the community. Nancy Mace, a nationally known educator, has been engaged to establish a training program for California Pacific Medical Center and the Alzheimer's Association of the Greater Bay Area.
Physical Environment *Description of setting*	The center is located in one of San Francisco's multicultural neighborhoods. The second floor of the Senior Services building is being renovated and will be devoted exclusively to the day and residential programs for patients with dementia. This space was originally designed as a traditional, triple-room nursing home. The final plan for renovation has decreased the institutional spatial effects of long corridors, double rooms, a dominant nursing station, and limited communal space despite the restrictions posed by regulatory codes, existing plumbing, and the location of bearing walls.
Description of the plan	The adult day care program will be housed at one end of the building and will be separated from the residential program. The two program areas surround a large outdoor space that provides opportunities for walking, gardening, or sitting. There is also a large garden area at the rear of the facility, which is available to residents accompanied by staff or volunteers. The residential unit is horseshoe shaped, with three small clusters of bedrooms. Communal and small group spaces are central to the unit. A gallery creates transitional space from the indoor living spaces to the outdoor patio.
Living space	Central to the living area is communal space that consists of two small activity/dining areas, a living room, and a porch. Adjoining each dining area is a small kitchen that allows residents to participate in food preparation and clean-up activities. Small dining areas support quiet, low-stress meals. Meals and supportive services will be provided by the Senior Services facility. Two activity rooms allow scheduling of concurrent activities to meet differing interests, while the larger living room provides a comfortable amount of space for larger group activities. Toilets adjoin both activity areas.

Toilet and bathing rooms

A sink and a toilet are provided in every resident's room, allowing prompt response to residents' needs. Shower facilities are located off the corridors.

Staff space

A small staff office and a staff lounge replace the traditional nurses' station. A conference room and resource library are also available for family conferences, staff meetings, training sessions, and caregiver support group meetings.

Equipment and furnishings

An interior designer with expertise in the needs of clients with dementia has been retained. Plans include the use of residential furnishings and finishes.

Corinne Dolan Alzheimer Center at Heather Hill

Address	12340 Bass Lake Road Chardon, OH 44024 (216) 942-6424
Owner	Heather Hill, Inc.
Staff contacts	Chari Weber, Vice President of Special Projects Kevan Namazi, Ph.D., Research Director
Facility type	The Corinne Dolan Alzheimer Center provides day, respite, and long-term care for people in the early and middle stages of dementia. It is situated on the grounds of a 234-bed, multidisciplinary, multilevel health care complex offering an extensive continuum of medical and rehabilitative services. The center is licensed as a rest home.
Residents	23 rest home residents, plus 6 to 10 day care clients and 1 respite bed
Staff	Director, program supervisors, health coordinator, program coordinators, and a research director and staff
Staff to resident ratio	1:6 direct care staff members
Site/context	Located on a 150-acre campus in rural Munson Township, 22 miles east of Cleveland, Ohio, the center extends the existing continuum of care at Heather Hill, which includes assisted living, intermediate and skilled nursing care, an existing nursing home unit for dementia care, and an acute rehabilitation hospital.
Size	14,000 square feet (approximate), exclusive of offices and the research department (2,250 square feet)
Date of completion	Fall 1989
Architect	Stephen Nemtim Taliesin Associated Architects of the Frank Lloyd Wright Foundation Scottsdale, Arizona The two-acre therapeutic park was developed in cooperation with the Holden Arboretum's Horticultural Therapy Department.
Sample publications	Epstein, N. (1988). Meeting needs of Alzheimer's patients. *American Medical News,* 11 March. Bowe, J. (1988). State-of-the-art Alzheimer's facilities take the lead in scientific research. *Today's Nursing Home, 8.* This analysis is based largely on staff self-reports.

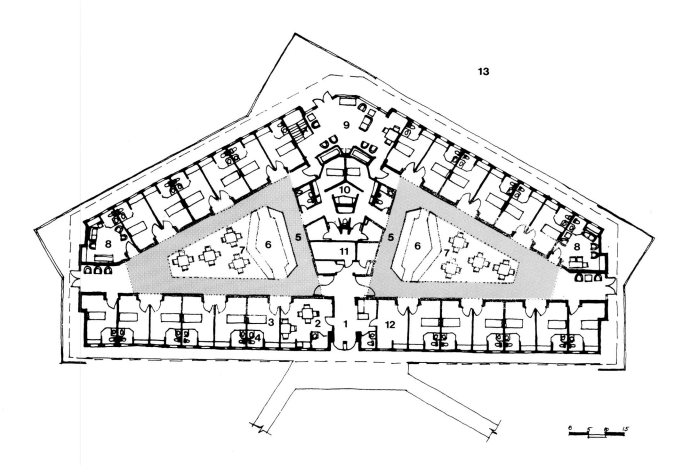

1   entry and reception area
2   crafts studio and day care entry
3   typical resident room
4   typical toilet area
5   wandering path
6   nourishment center (kitchen)
7   dining area
8   activity room/family room/lounge
9   living room
10 tub and shower rooms
11 support areas
12 offices
13 two-acre outdoor park

Variety of Activity Alcoves

+   The building offers a large number of activity spaces: the central public and dining areas (7); activity rooms (8); a living room (9); and a crafts studio (2). In addition, the wandering path, terrace, and outdoor park add to the range of places for activities. These places vary in size, location, and atmosphere; some are intimate and private, and others are stimulating and public. The number and variety of spaces for activities allow simultaneous programming for individuals and groups.

Noninstitutional Environment

The interior public space is large and differs from common residential dining and living rooms. This space is decorated in a "country-kitchen" motif and is used primarily for dining, food-related activities, and informal social interaction.

+   The incorporation of staff support spaces into the "domestic" elements of the environment helps to deinstitutionalize the unit. Staff members use the serving kitchen as a work and control point; there is no formal nurses' station, and other support areas are placed in a central but discreet location, with minimal exposure to the public domain.

—   The size and configuration of the large open space can, at times, overwhelm some residents; there are few windows with views to the outside, which may lead to disorientation. The clerestory windows allow some light into the facility, but its distribution is uneven.

Positive and Secure Outdoor Space

+   The outdoor park and the overall site has a secure, unobtrusive perimeter boundary; this allows totally free involvement of residents throughout the unit, the building, and the outdoors (weather permitting). The building has electronic controls on exterior doors, which can be locked in bad weather.

Secure Indoor Space

+   Interior doors to restricted areas, such as the housekeeping area, have push-button locks.

Personalization of the Environment

+   In addition to common strategies often used to provide a measure of personalization (e.g., bringing a piece of furniture from home), the center is experimenting with several design elements, such as the glass display case near the door to residents' rooms, for the display of personal items. A second strategy is the open shelving installed in residents' wardrobes, to be used as appropriate for each individual.

Research and Demonstration Site

The Corinne Dolan Alzheimer Center was conceived and planned as a research and assessment center. The identical organization of the two households and the experimental structure of the toilet rooms are some of the physical features of the research program.

Background
History

Heather Hill is a nonprofit, nonsectarian, extensive continuum of care campus located in rural Chardon, Ohio. It was one of the first long-term care facilities in the United States to establish a unit specifically for the care of people with dementia. A section of the nursing home was dedicated for this purpose in 1981.

The development process

In 1985, planning began to evaluate the needs of people with Alzheimer's disease and their families and to assess currently available programs and environments. The planning stage was funded by the Robert Wood Johnson Foundation. The results of these studies inspired the Dolan Family Foundation of Oyster Bay, New York, to award a major grant for the construction of the Alzheimer Center, which is named in honor of the late Corinne Dolan of Cleveland Heights.

A prominent architectural firm without extensive experience building nursing homes was selected to discourage traditional, institutional, or medical-model design.

Mission

The mission of the center is to develop model care programs and investigate ways of improving the quality of life for people with Alzheimer's disease and their families.

Funding

The cost of constructing, landscaping, equipping, and furnishing the center totaled approximately $3.5 million. The Dolan Family Foundation contributed $2.5 million for construction in addition to other gifts and grants, including funds for the therapeutic park. The Cleveland Foundation provided initial funding for the research department. Nearly $1 million—the balance of the funds needed to complete the project—was obtained from local and national foundations and corporations and from individuals.

Current costs (1992)

- Day care: Day care participants pay $30 for eight hours and $20 for four hours.
- Respite: Overnight respite residents pay $120 per night.
- Residential care: Long-term care residents pay $102 per day, with additional fees for pharmaceuticals, supplies, and physicians' services.

As an assisted living facility, the Corinne Dolan Alzheimer Center is not certified by the Department of Human Services as a Medicaid provider.

Services

The center is located on the campus of the Heather Hill continuum of care complex, which provides access to additional services, including a podiatrist and a dentist.

Education

The Corinne Dolan Alzheimer Center encourages the professional exchange of care-giving information and experiences. Educational conferences, a resource center, internships, and the studies and publications of the research department are aimed at the educational development of staff, family caregivers, and personnel from other facilities. Educational forums, seminars, and workshops are held regularly on topics of interest to audiences ranging from families and caregivers to medical and health care professionals.

Research

The mission, program, and design of the center reflect its dedication to research on AD. Examples of the types of issues researched include studies of disorientation, incontinence, distractability, confusion, nutritional deficiency, and the reinstating of familiar tasks. The emphasis of research is on behavioral problems and environmental solutions.

Goals
Key therapeutic goals

- *Provide a noninstitutional environment* (e.g., minimal use of carts, food service in a family style, absence of a paging system).
- *Provide opportunities for personalization* (e.g., provision of private bedrooms that residents furnish themselves, adoption of display cases outside residents' rooms to house personal momentos).
- *Provide opportunities for control and self-determination* (e.g., freedom to go outside to the park, resident control of the HVAC system, access to coffee and snacks as desired, freedom to wake up or go to sleep at any desired time).
- *Provide environmental opportunities for a variety of social interactions* (e.g., small sitting spaces for one or two, small group activity/visiting rooms, large group activity spaces).
- *Create secure freedom* (e.g., freedom to go outside, environmentally controlled access to off-limit areas).

Organizational goals

- *Advance research.* Both the building and the program are designed as prototypical, demonstration models, specifically for the support of systematic, empirical research.

Organizational and Social Environment
The staff

Positions and Ratios

Staff members include a director, program supervisors, a health coordinator, and program coordinators. A research director and staff are also an integral part of the care team.

Organizational Structure and Staffing

The center is composed of two identical units with twelve beds in each, plus common spaces shared by residents and day and respite care participants.

Training

All staff hired by the facility must have no recent nursing home experience— or none at all. Two-week orientation sessions include extensive education about Alzheimer's disease, as well as discussion of topics such as how to use the physical environment as a care-giving tool.

Characteristics of the Residents

The long-term care program currently includes twenty-three residents, plus additional day and respite care clients. All residents are ambulatory.

Admission and Retention

Applicants must receive approval from their family physician to be admitted as a respite or long-term resident, as the Corinne Dolan Alzheimer Center is a supportive residential model, not a nursing home. Applicants must have a diagnosis of probable Alzheimer's disease and must be ambulatory. All residents receive a preadmission assessment, including interviews and discussion with the caregiver, family, resident, and center staff. A complete geriatric evaluation may be required. Applicants are encouraged to participate in day care and/or night respite visits before admission. Priority is given to local residents and to those applicants who have previously attended the center.

Respite visits usually last three days to three weeks. Most day care participants attend on a regularly scheduled basis, and minimum participation is a four-hour visit. Day care is offered seven days a week. Advance application and scheduling are required. Participants may require only limited supervision from staff or may require help with almost all daily needs; however, applicants requiring skilled nursing care are not accepted. Participants who are self-destructive or who require physical or chemical restraint are not maintained in the program.

Residents requiring intensive medical care may be transferred to a step-down unit in the adjacent long-term care facility.

Program Description

Residents (and day and respite care participants) are assigned to small, family-style groups for most of their daily routine. The needs of each resident are assessed, and an individual plan is developed in which the resident is assigned to one of four program options. The first of these, the *community circle,* is a fairly high-intensity but comfortable routine of structured programs and activities, involving group social interactions, cooperation, and mental stimulation. Such activities include discussion groups, sports, crafts, and lifelong learning classes. The *family circle* is a home-structured program based primarily on familiar, past life events, enhancing residents' continuity with the past and sense of security and productivity. It includes activities such as laundry, cooking, shop work, and housekeeping. The *open circle* is a flexible structured program that meets the needs of residents with very limited abilities to focus attention or to communicate. It is also directed to very restless or reclusive residents. The building and program are design to provide walking spaces and activity nooks for such residents. Music groups, parties, simple games and exercises, and individual discussion and projects are offered at this level. The *men's club* is a program that focuses on traditional "masculine" chores and outings. Simple maintenance projects, yard and garden work, sports, and exercise are all offered in this option.

A variety of outings are scheduled for each program option, and family members are welcome to participate. A daily program is planned for each resident as part of the preadmission assessment, which is reviewed on a regular basis. Residents may move from one option to another as their needs or abilities change. Consistent staff assignments are maintained with each group.

Physical Environment
Description of the plan

The Corinne Dolan Alzheimer Center is a single-story structure composed of two triangular units with a shared support and bathing core. The open plan of each twelve-bed unit allows staff easy visual access to all participants and provides a continuous path for wanderers. Each unit has a fully equipped, residential-style kitchen/activity center, with generous counter and work space, a dining room, and a program/activity room.

In addition, there is a craft/activity room near the main entrance, which was designed to allow day care participants to enter and leave without being detected by other residents. There is also a central living room with a fireplace that serves both units.

Principles of spatial arrangement

Household

Rooms for twelve residents define a family cluster or "household."

Family Commons

At the center of each cluster is a shared living, dining, and cooking area (fig. 2.11).

Figure 2.11
The family commons is a center of activity in each household. (Photo by Maggie Calkins.)

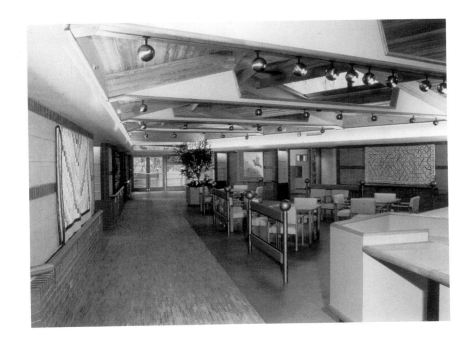

Wandering Path

The perimeters of the common areas provide a continuous loop for wandering.

Outdoor spaces

The goals of the outdoor design were to provide color year-round and to ensure a variety of different experiences in four primary activity areas: a wild flower field near the entrance drive; a natural area with seating and a view of the brook; an activity patio with seating and raised planters for gardening; and wandering gardens designed for rest, observation of nature, and various activities.

The upper patio, adjacent to the walkway, has chairs and tables overlooking the rest of the garden. The gently sloping path leads to a program center, where picnic tables are arranged. Residents can also pull chairs up to the circular garden wall to garden without stooping. Circular paths lead through the woods to scenic views and to grassy areas where residents play croquet and practice putting. All paths circle back to the main path in the center to aid in wayfinding.

Special efforts were made to shield distracting views and to ensure wheelchair accessibility. Lighting is geared for both day and evening activities. In general, outdoor security is intended to be unobtrusive. Exit doors are equipped with an access control device, unlocked during clement weather to provide residents with open access to the park. The two-acre outdoor area includes over ninety species of nontoxic plants.

A variety of additional activity areas are planned, including a flag pole, clothes line, hand pump, and small playground for children.

Wandering path

Adjacent to each resident room doorway is an interior walking path, surrounding the kitchen and dining areas. The plan of the facility eliminates all dead-end corridors. The wandering path is differentiated from the adjacent area by a change in floor materials (from carpet or resilient floor to hardwood floors in circulation spaces).

Living rooms and social spaces

The household plan of the each unit is complemented by a family room, used for small group activities and visiting. For research purposes, both family rooms are identical in shape, decor, and respective location. A large living room with a fireplace and a view of the surrounding landscape is used as an additional meeting place for residents and families. Several small nooks are also designated for casual conversation and visiting. These are located adjacent to the exits, where they are clearly visible to staff members.

Kitchen/dining areas

A residential-style kitchen is one of the focal points of each unit, intended to encourage residents to continue familiar, domestic patterns. Work space is provided at both counter and table heights to allow residents to stand or sit while working. The kitchens can be closed off to allow staff members to prepare meals safely and efficiently or can be opened for general participation. Healthy snacks are available for residents at all times.

Adjacent to the kitchen is the dining area (fig. 2.12). The wheelchair-accessible matte surface tables here are designed to fit together in different configurations to accommodate groups of one to six residents. The barriers between the dining rooms and the halls are designed to be flexible to test the effects of different types of barriers. Residents can easily watch ongoing activities or socialize in the dining area.

Figure 2.12
The central kitchen dining area in each unit serves as a focal point for residents' activity. Partitions in these areas are flexible to allow reearch on wayfinding and distractabilty. (Photo by Maggie Calkins.)

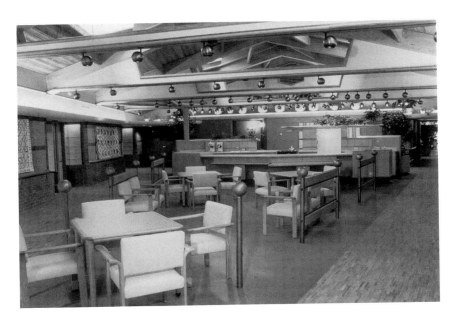

Activity rooms

In addition to the kitchen, dining room, and family room in each unit and the shared living room, a crafts room provides residents with the opportunity to participate in various projects, including painting and woodworking.

Residents' rooms

Private bedrooms are arranged around the perimeter of the wandering path. Dutch doors on bedrooms allow exterior orientation and additional natural light into the central area and at the same time maintain privacy and discourage rummaging in residents' rooms. Each bedroom has a locked display case at the entrance to hold the resident's treasured mementos. This case is intended as a secure place for items of value and as an orientation cue relying on remote memory to help residents find their respective rooms. The display cases also offer personal insight about the resident to other residents and staff members. Each resident has a private room with a large, curved, picture window overlooking the rustic outdoors. Residents are encouraged to furnish their own rooms with furnishings from home.

Toilet and shower/ tub rooms

Within each resident room, a toilet is located along an exterior wall, where it is clearly visible but can be shielded by a wrap-around curtain when in use

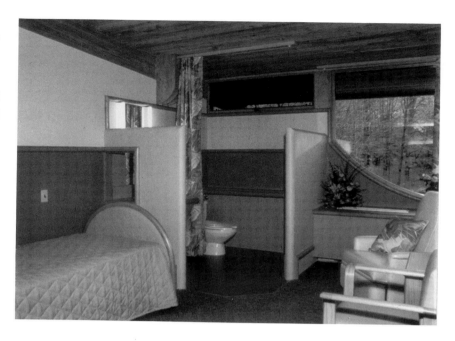

Figure 2.13
Visible toilets in residents' rooms are intended to increase residents' ease in locating and remembering to use toilets. Surrounding curtains can be pulled to provide visual privacy when in use. (Photo by Maggie Calkins.)

(fig. 2.13). This strategy is intended to make the toilet more visible, aiding the resident in locating and remembering to use it.

A common bathing area is located in the core of the facility, to be shared by residents of both units. Bathroom fixtures resemble conventional home tubs and showers; a whirlpool is also available.

Equipment and furnishings

Although primarily of residential style, a number of different furnishings (including chairs, tables, bathtubs, door handles, and faucets) have been tested for their effectiveness with this population. Residents bring all furniture and other belongings to personalize their room.

Primary room light is provided by an uplighting system, intended to decrease glare.

Wall hangings along the wandering paths consist of washable quilts and tactile paintings to encourage residents to explore their environment both visually and tactilely.

Materials and surfaces

The interior public walls are brick from the floor to the railing and blasted concrete block above. The circulation zone has hardwood floors, and other areas have either resilient flooring or carpeting (several varieties have been tested). Some rooms are designed to accommodate both carpet and resilient flooring to test the suitability of each for this population.

Friendship House, Cedar Lake Home Campus

Address	5595 Highway Z West Bend, WI 53095 (414) 334-9487
Owner	Benevolent Corporation of the Cedar Lake Home Campus (nonprofit, United Church of Christ affiliate)
Staff contact	Donna Kehle, Resident Family Service Coordinator
Facility type	Freestanding long-term care facility intentionally designed for people with dementia, located within a large continuum of care
Residents	Total of 128, arranged in eight households of 16 residents each; stages 1 and 2
Staff	16 nurses' aides and 2 nurses. An activity coordinator, a music therapist, a social worker, a nursing supervisor, and a director of nursing are shared with Fellowship House, a skilled care nursing home.
Staff to resident ratio	Approximately 1:7
Site/context	245-acre campus, which includes independent housing, retirement housing, an education/retreat center, day care, rehabilitation, housing for people with dementia, and a skilled care nursing home facility. The Cedar Lake Home Campus is located five miles from West Bend, Wisconsin.
Size (approximate square footage)	3,388 square feet/household unit 27,104 square feet/residential floor (eight units) 49,462 square feet/total building
Date of completion	March 1976
Architects	Guerin & Mooney, Milwaukee, Wisconsin

The description of this facility pertains to Friendship House as it was planned and conceived and as it was operated between 1976 and approximately 1989. Because of changes in the resident population and in administrative philosophy, a new facility is currently being constructed on the Cedar Lake Home Campus to accommodate people with Alzheimer's disease. The design principles and therapeutic objectives of this new facility are not necessarily similar to (or compatible with) those described here. The current Friendship House building will remain intact after the transfer of its residents to the new facility; however, Friendship House will serve another population in the future.

Figure 2.14   Plan of the Friendship House, Cedar Lake Home Campus, West Bend, Wisconsin.

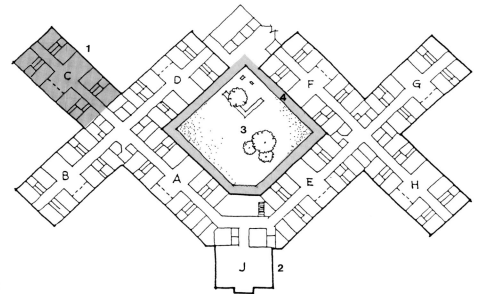

1   typical household (*C*), one of eight units
2   entry at lower level
3   secure outdoor yard
4   outdoor wandering path

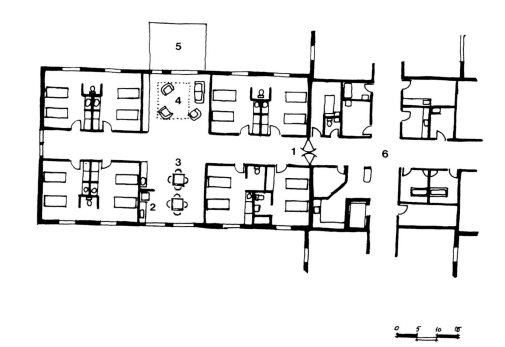

1   entry
2   serving kitchen
3   dining/activity area
4   living room
5   patio
6   service core

Small Groups of Residents

+ This facility is credited as one of the pioneering attempts to establish the "family cluster" or "household" concept. The solution is simple but elegant: the living room and kitchen/dining room, along with the partial elimination of the long corridor, create a domestic core for each group of eight rooms.

Continuum of Care

+ The building comprises of eight identical households, which allows clustering of residents according to their needs and abilities. The facility also allows aging in place—continuing service to the same residents as their needs change over time.

Positive Outdoor Space

+ The geometry of the building creates a protected outdoor space without the use of an obtrusive fence. The courtyard is directly accessible from four households.

− The wandering path is too close to the surrounding bedroom windows.

Internal Circulation

− The building's organization—two identical X forms with mirror image symmetry—gives rise to potentially confusing and disorienting paths with many undifferentiated intersections.

− Certain households (*A* and *E*) are at the distinct disadvantage of serving as a passageway for all other units.

− Unlike the outdoor wandering path, which is clear and continuous, the internal path is interrupted by several dead-end closures.

Background
History

The Cedar Lake Home Campus is one of three Cedar Lake campuses in south-eastern Wisconsin, along with Cedar Ridge (a retirement community) and Cedar Valley (a retreat campus). Owned by the Benevolent Corporation of the Cedar Lake Home Campus, the 245-acre Cedar Lake Home Campus is a continuum of care community located five miles from West Bend, thirty-five miles northwest of Milwaukee.

The development process

Friendship House, completed in March 1976, was the first freestanding U.S. facility intended expressly for people with Alzheimer's and related disorders. The following discussion describes Friendship House as it was planned, conceived, and operated between 1976 and approximately 1989. In recent years, the facility has witnessed a change in its resident population, from many residents in the early stages of the disease, still fairly cognitively intact, toward a population of residents almost all of whom are in the advanced stages of the disease with more severe, dementia-related impairments. Administrators hypothesize that this change may be due to the increasing number of options available in the region for maintaining the person with dementia in the community for an extended period (e.g., day care, respite care, and community-based group homes), with the resultant effect that the typical person with dementia does not enter a facility such as Friendship House until he or she has reached an advanced stage of the disease.

For this (and perhaps other reasons), the current resident population of Cedar Lake is more severely impaired than the population in residence when the facility was planned and designed in the early 1970s. Many design and policy innovations intended to benefit a less-impaired population are no longer appropriate or effective, in the opinion of the administration. (However, it is quite possible that a more impaired dementia population might continue to benefit from therapeutic design interventions other than those originally intended for the original, less-impaired population.) Management priorities also appear to have shifted toward increased concern for the convenience of the staff in maintenance and care. In any case, these changes have necessitated the construction of a new facility for people with dementia on the campus, adjacent to Friendship House. The current Friendship House building will remain intact after construction of the new facility; however, Friendship House is intended to serve another population in the future; it may be renovated into community-based group homes. The design principles, therapeutic objectives, and actual design of the new building are not necessarily similar to those described here.

Services

The Cedar Lake Home Campus includes day care and rehabilitation services, independent and assisted living housing, educational and social services, a skilled care nursing home, and Friendship House, a freestanding facility for people with Alzheimer's disease. Two separate facilities—an apartment complex for retired persons located three miles away and an education/retreat center located fifteen miles to the north—are also affiliated with the main campus.

Goals
Key therapeutic goals

- *Stabilize residents' condition.* Reduce the anxiety, agitation, and potential confusion of new residents.
- *Maintain independence and purpose.* Contribute to an active, independent life with a sense of purpose.
- *Minimize or eliminate medication and restraint.*
- *Maintain normalcy.* Attempt to preserve what is "normal" and familiar to residents in the physical environment. Policies that encourage the inclusion of furnishings from home in residents' rooms reinforce this goal, as do design features such as household kitchenettes that support familiar kitchen-related activities from the past.
- *Promote positive feelings among family members.* Seriously consider the needs of family members; provide a comfortable, familiar, nonthreatening environment that offers "things to do" and to talk about during visiting. Many attributes of the facility, such as the pool table in the first floor conversation corner and the spinning wheel and other conversation pieces in public social areas, were added to the facility with this goal in mind.

Organizational and Social Environment
The staff

Positions and Ratios

Two aides are assigned to each of the eight households, and one nurse serves every four households. A registered nurse is on duty twenty-four hours a day. Specialized services and upper level management are supplemented by campus-wide resources (e.g., music therapy, social worker).

Training

Friendship House maintains its own in-house training program for nursing aides to instill Cedar Lake's philosophies, policies, and procedures from the beginning of staff members' experience with elderly persons and people with dementia.

The residents

Characteristics of the Residents

Friendship House serves a total of 128 residents, arranged in eight households of 16 residents each.

Program Description

The structured and flexible program provides regular and predictable activities, at the same time allowing residents choice regarding participation (e.g., beauty shop, music room, German club).

Physical Environment
Description of the plan

The building is constructed on a sloping site. The ground floor includes the entry zone and all major support services; most of these spaces are subterranean. Such spaces include laundry facilities, an employee lounge and separate employee cafeteria, and the primary facility kitchen.

The residential portion of Friendship House, on the first floor, comprises two clusters of four households each. A nurse's station, elevator, and services are located at the center of each cluster of four households. An auditorium/dining area is located at the junction of the two clusters.

Principles of spatial arrangement

One of the unique and original characteristics of Cedar Lake is its arrangement into separate households intended to function at the "family" scale in terms of both physical design and programmatic features. Each household includes eight double rooms; in most cases, two resident rooms (and four residents) share a bathroom. At the center of each household are a "living room" and a "dining room/kitchenette," located to either side of the central corridor. All residents eat in a common, central dining room, with the exception of those residents unable to feed themselves. (This is perhaps a missed opportunity for small group interaction in a facility designed around household-based kitchenettes and dining areas.) These residents are fed in the households. The central dining room is also used for large group activities, such as meetings of the resident German club and chapel services.

Entry area

The ground floor front lobby—Friendship House's main entrance—contains homelike furnishings, interesting conversational objects (e.g., a spinning wheel and holiday decorations), paintings by a local artist, and display cases filled with crafts completed by residents of Friendship House and other units.

Figure 2.15
Cedar Lake includes many social spaces for visiting with residents on the ground and second floors, complete with conversation pieces and "things to do" to encourage social interaction while visiting. This unique mounted flying fish was contributed by a resident of the facility. It now serves as an important landmark for residents and as a conversation stimulus.

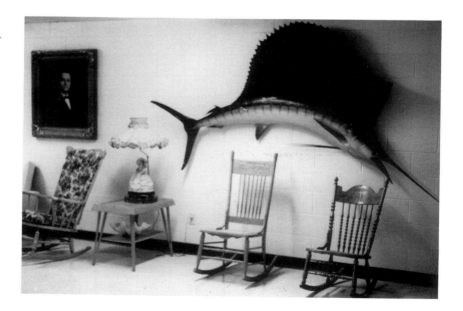

These items are intended to serve as stimuli for conversation between residents and visitors and to reinforce a noninstitutional ambience (fig. 2.15). The lobby area more closely resembles a rustic country lodge than a traditional nursing home. However, there is some debate among staff members as to whether the lobby should be more "presentable" and less "homelike."

The hallways of the ground floor are lined with paintings by a resident of Friendship House, who began to paint with staff encouragement after entering the facility. These paintings serve as a stimulus for conversation, according to staff members, as visitors and residents frequently identify with the familiar scenes from the painter's life growing up in southeastern Wisconsin.

Museum

A former storage room on the lower level has been transformed into a museum with an extensive collection of furnishings and artifacts provided by residents and their families (fig. 2.16). The museum is a potentially effective

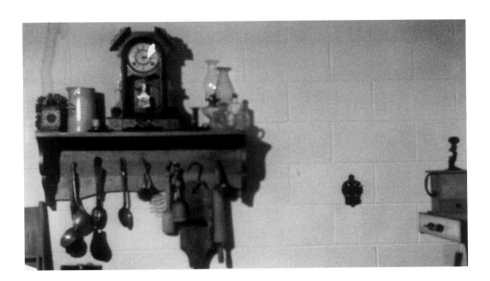

Figure 2.16
This museum of personal belongings is a rich addition to the facility. Even residents who cannot remember recent events may recall significant aspects of their own past when viewing objects from the museum. In addition, the ability to store personal objects in the museum assures residents that their important belongings will be cared for and appreciated.

trigger for reminiscence and a popular destination for visiting. However, residents' actual access to the museum is quite limited. Administrators also find the museum overstimulating to residents. (A more even distribution of the museum artifacts throughout the facility might encourage more frequent resident contact with and recognition of these items from their pasts.)

Outdoor spaces

Outdoors, the geometry of the building creates a protected, inner, donut-shaped outdoor space without the necessity of fencing. This space is directly accessible from half of the units. The outdoor area is popular as a destination when visiting with residents. Several trees provide shade for residents relaxing on benches and at patio chairs around tables.

A wooden planter—raised about thirty inches above grade—is the focus of gardening activities when weather permits. In a corner structure, several fenced bins house animals during the summer.

This central, grassy courtyard is surrounded by a wandering path. (The location of the wandering path on the periphery of the outdoor space, directly adjacent to the windows of the residents' rooms, is potentially problematic, as wandering residents may cast shadows on the windows and disturb or alarm residents indoors.)

Direct access to the outdoors is provided from four of the households (a positive aspect of this space, although one might feel "on display" while in the courtyard). Units that do not have direct access to the outdoors are those occupied by residents in more advanced stages of the disease. These units have views to a natural wooded area behind the facility, reminiscent of the rural landscape that may be familiar to those residents from the region.

Wandering path

Residents wander within the individual households. One administrator reported that the short, dead-end corridors are preferable to a continuous "race track," as residents feel a sense of accomplishment in reaching a destination.

Kitchenette/living/ dining area

Flexible living/dining areas with kitchenettes are created in each household by borrowing space from the corridor (fig. 2.17). The fully equipped kitchenettes are complete with refrigerators and ovens, which can be controlled at the breaker box. (Surface units are removed in households with more impaired residents.)

Unusual, ceiling-mounted, upward-folding tables have been permanently installed in household dining areas and in dining and meeting areas throughout the facility. These tables were selected for their performance along several criteria: wheelchair accessibility, ease of putting them away when not in use to save space in common areas, and ease of cleaning. (Unfortunately, the strange appearance of the tables greatly increases the unfamiliar, institutional nature of these spaces—the tables could not be considered "normal" according to almost any standards. In addition, the fixed location of the tables disallows flexibility in table arrangement to accommodate changes in function of the spaces.)

A small, informal table used for charting and paperwork replaces the tradi-

Figure 2.17
The domestic kitchen in each household provides a locus for activity (beverage making, snack preparation, etc.), adds to the domestic character of the household, and serves as a catalyst for social activities of residents and caregivers.

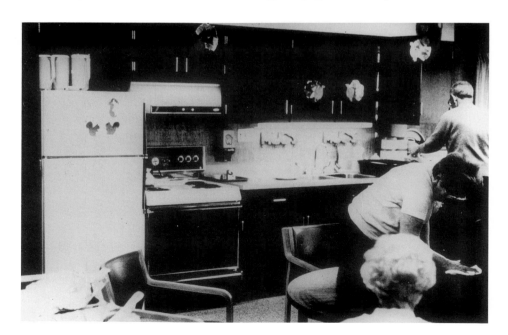

tional, fortress-like nursing station. The absence of a nurse's station significantly deinstitutionalizes the character of the household.

Residents' rooms

All residents' rooms are designed to accommodate two residents. While this arrangement is less expensive than the provision of single rooms for all residents, double rooms are also perceived by administrators as helpful for combating resident withdrawal. Residents' rooms house a mix of traditional nursing home furnishings (e.g., hospital beds) and selected personal items (e.g., dressers from home). Curtains are provided for all windows in residents' rooms.

Vinyl floor surfaces continue into residents' rooms. (Carpeting in residents' rooms is not recommended; in the opinion of administrators, its appearance is difficult to maintain over time.) Many residents' rooms are marked outside by familiar, personal mementos contributed by family members. Administrators report that recognizable, individualized cues seem to be most successful in helping residents to locate their own rooms.

Toilet and shower/ tub rooms

Toilet rooms are located between every two resident rooms for use by a total of four residents. Staff members feel that the small size and the configuration of these spaces make them inconvenient for use by residents who require assistance when toileting (an increasing percentage of the residents of Friendship House).

Staff "retreat" and lounge areas

A designated lounge for staff retreat is located on the ground floor, away from the residential households above. A separate staff cafeteria is also provided, as staff members are not permitted to eat in the lounge. A formal and separate area for staff retreat is perceived by staff members as critical, given the recent trend toward increased impairment in the resident population, who now demand more intensive nursing care of staff members. Because of increased demands on staff time and patience in the household, distinct areas for staff retreat and dining are deemed necessary and important for respite from the demands of the household. In addition, due to the questionable ability of residents to engage in social interaction with staff, the maintenance of a separate area for staff meals and retreat does not constitute a lost opportunity for staff/ resident interaction (in the opinion of staff members).

Equipment and furnishings

Furnishings in living/dining rooms are institutional in character, comprising largely built-ins with vinyl and dark laminate surfaces. In a makeshift response to resident incontinence in households occupied by residents in advanced stages of dementia, all living/dining room chairs are covered with rubber sheets and pads at all times. (Although this solution increases the ease of cleaning up after accidents, it detracts from the residential nature of the household, and, when employed alone, it does not decrease the incidence of incontinence, nor does it improve residents' feelings of competence or staff members' morale or attitudes toward residents.)

Seasonal decorations are incorporated into the households, enhancing their homelike and familiar image for residents. Decorations are intended to respond to the level of competence of the residents; for example, poinsettias and decorated Christmas trees are allowed in households where residents will not ingest them.

Doors into households can be locked or left open. If locked, staff members and visitors can enter the household but must unlock the door to leave. Views to other households through windows in the doors seem undesirable, but staff members do not see this as a problem. Rooms used only occasionally (e.g., music room, beauty shop) are kept locked when not is use.

Materials and surfaces

Vinyl flooring is used throughout the households, with carpeted wainscotting on corridor walls. Walls are painted cinder block in most areas. Nevertheless, a homelike atmosphere emerges despite the relatively institutional materials and surfaces. The small social and physical scale of the household seems very successful in this regard. The relatively small scale of the household may constitute a potential compromise, in that this design pre-empts the possibility of any long interior paths for wandering.

Minna Murra Lodge

Address	25 Stenner Street P.O. Box 815 Toowoomba, Queensland 4350, Australia 6176-35 8279
Owner	Toowoomba Garden Settlement, an agency of the Uniting Church in Australia Property Trust (Q)
Staff contacts	Ms. Merle Perring O.A.M., Chief Executive Officer Barry Whisson, Architect
Facility type	Freestanding group home facility specifically designed for people with dementia who wander; located within a large campus of continuum of care
Residents	15 residents; 14 positions for long-term residents, and 1 for respite care
Staff	A hospital supervisor, personal care attendants, and program assistants provide direct care for residents. Therapists and a hairdresser, podiatrist, optometrist, and chaplain—all from the continuum of care complex—are also available to residents. Administration is provided by staff from the head office.
Staff to resident ratio	1:4 from 7:00 a.m. to 6:30 p.m.; 1:5 from 6:30 p.m. to 10:30 p.m.; 1:15 from 10:30 p.m. to 7:00 a.m. An additional staff member lives in the attached staff accommodation and is on call for emergency situations.
Site/context	A 30-acre complex located in suburban Toowoomba (population 90,000), less than two miles from the central business district. The total population of the complex is 161 residents. The range of care comprises standard hostels, independent living units, nursing home care, a day therapy center for rehabilitation, day care, home care services, and the Minna Murra Lodge.
Size	Approximately 8,000 square feet of a total 13,000 square foot roofed area; single story, all on one level
Date of completion	June 1986
Architects	Downs Designed Environments Pty. Ltd., Barry J. Whisson, B. Arch, A.R.A.I.A., director and designer

This analysis is based largely on the architect's and the chief executive officer's self-reports.

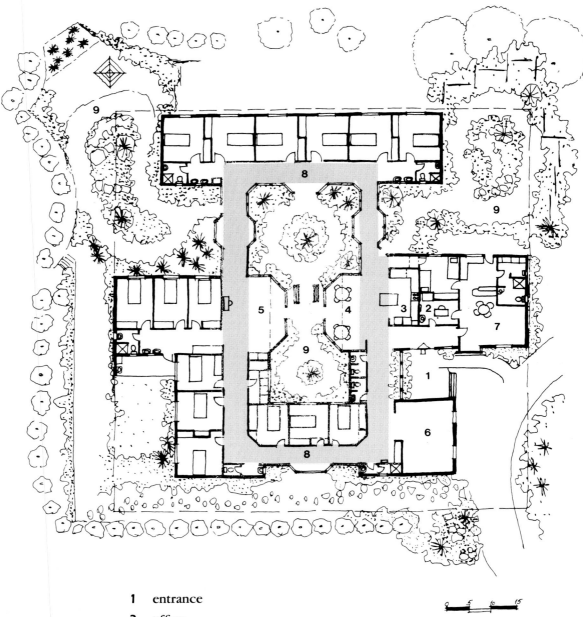

1   entrance
2   office
3   kitchen
4   dining room
5   activity area
6   lounge
7   auxiliary apartment
8   wandering path
9   secure courtyard

Meaningful Wandering Path

+ The wandering path (8) that surrounds the interior courtyard (9) is an integral part of the public space of the facility. It includes activity nooks and rest places, thus facilitating either continuous wandering or participation in an activity. Doors are minimized, eliminating the necessity to make numerous choices. The external outdoor yards (9) also have a circuitous path.

Positive Outdoor Space

+ The central outdoor courtyard (9) is the major organizing element in the unit's plan: it provides daylight and outdoor views to all internal spaces and aids in wayfinding and orientation.
+ The internal courtyard is secure, always open and accessible; it can accommodate both formal and informal activities.
+ The external outdoor yards (9) support various activity areas—from spaces for clothes drying to resting areas.

Noninstitutional Image

+ The overall design approach is to provide a house form akin to neighboring houses. The pitched roof, the building size, and the landscaping are all residential in character.
+ The building organization diminishes the institutional images through the minimization of corridors. There is no formal nurses' station, and the domestic features of the kitchen, dining room and living room are integrated with the public wandering path.
— The extensive use of the interior court and the wandering path results in a very dispersed plan, which lacks the intimacy of a house. The dining room (4) and kitchen (3) are not associated with the residential clusters and seem remote and public.

Background

History

Toowoomba Garden Settlement is a continuum of care complex comprising seven levels of care for the elderly; it has been in operation as a care entity since 1959. The complex is located in the suburbs of the city of Toowoomba, approximately eighty miles southwest of Brisbane, the capital of the state of Queensland. Minna Murra Lodge—a freestanding group home for fifteen people with dementia—was intended to serve as a complement to the existing facilities within the complex.

The property on which the complex is sited is vested in the Uniting Church in Australia Property Trust (Q). Although located in suburban Toowoomba, the complex enjoys a rural outlook, being bounded on one side by a park, on another by a market farming venture operated by a foundation for the mentally handicapped, and on a third side by commercial market farming.

Mission

Minna Murra Lodge was commissioned because, although accommodations were available for persons with mild dementia in standard hostels on the site, the organization had no facility for persons with moderate to severe dementia who were wanderers. Many caregivers had reached extreme crisis situations and the Board of Management responded to this need, commissioning the design and construction of a secure environment that addressed these issues. The organization's mission was strictly defined as the provision of a homelike environment for persons in the more advanced stages of dementia—persons who are ambulatory yet wanderers.

The essential design process fell under the direct control of the architect, who arranged ad hoc meetings, usually on a one-to-one basis, with team members. Because little information was available on designing for dementia at this time, extensive preparation was undertaken by the architect to understand and accommodate the needs of this population. The client (represented by various individuals and subgroups) was also a very active contributor to the design and development of the facility.

Funding

Funding was provided by three sources: the commonwealth government provided a building subsidy that met approximately half the cost of construction, the state government provided a subsidy toward furnishings (Australian $1250 per bed), and the balance was met from the organization's own resources.

Services

Minna Murra Lodge provides both long-term care and respite care for one overnight resident at a time.

Current status: accommodating changes in the resident population and in the context of care

The mission—to provide for wanderers in the moderate to late stages of AD—remains essentially the same as when the facility first opened. However, changes in the population of people with dementia and in the availability of care have prompted new development in the complex. First, more community options are now available to caregivers than when the lodge first opened. Because of this change, residents tend to remain in the community for a longer time before entering the facility and are consequently more physically frail on admission and have more severe behavioral problems than in the past. In addition, there is a greater demand for placement in the facility now than earlier, intensifying the sense of mission that drives the organization. This demand has created a new need to provide yet another facility for those both mentally and physically frail, with a different range of design parameters to be addressed; this facility, known as Epworth Nursing Home (with a linked special care unit), was completed and occupied in 1992.

Goals
Key therapeutic goals

- *Assist residents in maintaining the highest level of functional ability* possible for as long as possible.
- *Enable residents to feel comfortable, enhance their feelings of peace and dignity*—their feeling of being secure and loved.
- *Encourage residents to participate in activities that give a sense of achievement.*
- *Minimize the use of medication and restraints.*
- *Improve self-esteem and the sense of well-being.*
- *Make visits of family members and friends enjoyable and reduce feelings of guilt* among caregivers.
- *Achieve actual and perceived safety and security* for residents and staff.

Organizational and Social Environment
The staff

Positions and Ratios

Minna Murra Lodge is directed by a full-time supervisor, who has wide experience in geriatric nursing and in the care of people with dementia. Six part-time personal care attendants work a total of twenty-seven hours a day. Five program assistants provide an additional thirteen hours a day of direct care. In addition, volunteers provide approximately three hours a day of assistance in activities. Administration of the lodge is provided by the staff of the head office. Staff members work as a team of caregivers rather than on the basis of delineation of duties.

Staffing Ratios

Day time—1:4 (including the supervisor, a personal care attendant, a program assistant, and a domestic aide) from 7:00 a.m. to 6:30 p.m; evening—1:5 (including two personal care attendants and a program assistant) from 6:30 p.m. to 10:30 p.m.; night time—1:15 (a personal care attendant) from 10:30 p.m. to 7:00 a.m. An additional staff member lives in the attached staff accommodation and is available on call for emergencies.

Training: Modify the Staff, not the Residents

Staff members are carefully chosen for their personal qualities, attitudes, and practical and relevant experience with people with dementia. They are trained specifically for the care of this population. For example, staff members are taught to be perceptive to the individual needs of the residents and to respond accordingly, realizing that behavioral problem solving depends upon the ability of staff members to learn rather than the ability of the resident to change.

Morale and Retention

With the exception of the supervisor, all staff members work on a part-time basis to prevent burn out. There has been very little staff turnover since the lodge opened; in fact, most of the present staff have worked at this facility for the five years since it was commissioned.

The residents

Characteristics of the Residents

The fifteen residents (fourteen long term and one respite) have ranged in age from fifty-five to over ninety years. All residents are ambulatory. Most are incontinent and on a management program.

Admission and Retention

Residents must have a diagnosed irreversible dementia (moderate to severe) and must be wanderers. Residents are most often referred by medical practitioners. The Geriatric Assessment Team is involved in preadmission assessment. Computed tomographic scans and pathological tests are also performed on all residents. Final assessment is made during the first four weeks of occupancy to ensure appropriate placement.

Residents remain in Minna Murra Lodge until intensive medical needs necessitate transfer to the nursing home (redesigned and presently being rebuilt) within the complex.

The families

Visitors participate in both informal social interaction, particularly in the interior courtyard, and programmed activities, most frequently those taking place in the activity room.

Program Description

The program of Minna Murra is developed around achievable and nondemanding activities in a relaxed social and physical environment. The daily routine revolves around familiar household activities (a basic dimension of the program)—a continuous flow of normal daily activities involving the resident where practical. Residents are gently encouraged to participate in activities and are provided with options. Specific activities include music therapy, games, food preparation, massage, grooming, exercise, outdoor activities and outings, current events, and organized, nonstimulating evening programs. Because a detailed social history of each resident is developed upon his or her admission to the lodge, the activity program can be tailored to reflect individual interests and preferences.

Physical Environment

Description of the plan

The macro plan is essentially a "square donut"—the "hole" being represented by the enclosed secure courtyard, around which the "home" is arranged. The home comprises bedrooms and common spaces off single-loaded corridors, the secure wandering path. Careful attention was paid to climatic orientation and to siting. The visual image to the community is low key, akin to familiar hipped-roof houses. The plan itself was located to meld within its surroundings, retain the essential original bushland setting, minimally disturb the landscape, and visually complement other facilities in the complex.

Within the plan, the juxtaposition of rooms was organized to reflect that with which the residents would be familiar in their own home. The wandering path traverses through common areas (or down one open side of the same), such as the kitchen, dining room, lounge, activity areas, and sitting areas, to facilitate social interaction. Care was taken to minimize necessary decision making; thus, doors were kept to a minimum.

Principles of spatial arrangement

The interior courtyard and its surrounding circuitous wandering path dictate the shape of the facility. These are complemented by the surrounding external courtyards. There has been an emphasis in the planning not to overdesign but to enable reasonably effective changes in decor as needs permit in the future, while retaining the basic spatial arrangement.

Entry area

The front door of the facility is wheelchair accessible and visible from within the complex from the lounge and the supervisor's office, yet internally placed off the wandering path. Design interventions intended to restrict wandering into the area include carpeting, low lighting levels, and disguise of the entry by continuing a section of handrail across the door. The door is controlled by an electronic alarm.

Outdoor spaces

The fully enclosed internal courtyard is secure day and night, and exits to the area are left unlocked at all times. The courtyard is the home of the house canary and pet dog. This space serves as an additional wandering area and as a popular place for visiting. Herbs and mint are grown outside the kitchen door and used in cooking for the facility. Plants within the space were chosen for minimum maintenance and to allow opportunities for sweeping leaves from the paths, a functional activity for residents.

Two external courtyards are formed by a cut into the slope of the site and by lattice screen backdrops to planting, overcoming the need to fence in an obvious manner. One of the external courtyards leads to the clothes-drying area, and the other includes a water feature. A third exterior courtyard is used for maintenance facilities and storage.

An integral part of the exterior design is that of its contrived canopy—both built and unbuilt—of pergolas, roof, and planting, intended to increase the sense of perceived security.

Wandering path

The internal wandering path is circuitous around the building. Both the internal and external courtyards also employ circuitous paths; all are interrelated, and most are interconnected and relate directly to the interior wandering path. Wandering paths were designed to subtly encourage both the direction of wandering and social interaction. For example, the truncated corners in junctions of right-angled corridors encourage residents to keep moving, while the placement of tables and chairs suggests places to rest or engage in activity along the path. Throughout the facility, doors are minimized to ease decision making for wandering residents. All options are clearly identified by signs.

Living rooms and social spaces

The living room/lounge is located to one side of the wandering path, within easy reach of the kitchen and dining room (as in residents' past homes). Variable-size spaces for socialization and activities were intentionally accommodated in the design of the facility, including the lounge, the activity area, and small three-seat bay windows off the wandering path.

Kitchen/dining areas

The kitchen forms the center of the residents' "home," with the kitchen table being the central feature. The kitchen cupboards and sink are familiar in design, as is the electronically protected stove and oven. A refrigerator with a

Figure 2.19
View from the dining room to the interior landscaped courtyard. This central space provides abundant natural light and attractive views to the outside. (Photo by Barry Whisson.)

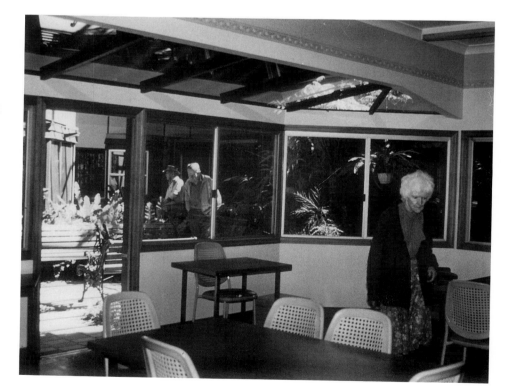

power outlet above residents' reach is also provided, together with a pantry alongside. The dining room is adjacent to the kitchen, across the wandering path. The kitchen/dining area is within visual and aural access of the activity area across the courtyard (fig. 2.19).

Activity room

A dedicated activity room includes versatile seating and table arrangements, access to a crafts and games cupboard, and a piano. Together with the lounge and kitchen/dining room, it accommodates concurrent programmed and unprogrammed activities. The activity space is most frequently utilized for evening activity programs.

Climatically, the location of the activity room was intended to maximize the advantages of cool summer breezes and warm winter sun—the latter through the glass roof annex that reinforces the image of this space as a conservatory, jutting out into the secure landscaped courtyard.

Residents' rooms

All bedrooms accommodate a single resident. These vary in size but are generally approximately 160 square feet, clear of built-in wardrobe space. Residents are encouraged to bring their own furniture, preferably a bedspread, a favorite chair, and/or a dressing table. Both locked and unlocked wardrobe space is provided in each resident's room (to control rummaging).

Flexibility in bedroom arrangement was designed into the plan. Modular wardrobes between adjacent single bedrooms can be removed and relocated to provide for couples if required. (Since the opening of the facility, there has not been a need to accommodate a couple.)

Toilet and shower/tub rooms

These are dispersed throughout the plan rather than attached to each resident room. The walking distance from bedrooms to bathrooms was carefully researched to accommodate this decision. Night lighting and light switches were coordinated with the placement of bathrooms.

Staff apartment and office

The supervisor's office faces the front entrance, from which entry and exit from the facility is informally monitored. The office is situated between the rest of the lodge and an auxiliary apartment for the supervisor, who serves as an on call aide in the event of nighttime emergencies. This apartment has a private patio (a portion of one of the external courtyards), kitchen, bedroom, bathroom, and living area. The door to the apartment is painted in the same color as the adjoining walls, and the quarters are soundproofed from the care unit itself.

Equipment and furnishings

Furnishings were selected to accommodate age deficits and allow practical upkeep. These have been supplemented by period furniture in keeping with the design of the facility. Familiar objects from the past (such as grandfather clocks), wooden handrails, natural fibers, and carefully chosen wall hangings are intended to reinforce the residential atmosphere and to serve as cues for wayfinding. Decoration is intended to provide low levels of stimulation and to ensure ease of maintenance.

Materials and surfaces

All surfaces and materials are intended to be easily maintainable and to reflect traditional styles of the region.

New Perspective Group Home #4

Address	11514 North Port Washington Road Mequon, WI (414) 241-9097
Owner	New Perspective
Staff contact	Suzanne Larson, President
Facility type	Freestanding community-based group home specially designed for people with dementia. This is one of five such group homes currently owned and operated by New Perspective in the Milwaukee area, with additional facilities under construction.
Residents	12, ranging from early stage 2 to stage 3 and including nonverbal and incontinent residents
Staff	Manager, assistant manager, and primary and secondary aides. An activity coordinator, massage therapist, and nutritionist operate among all five homes (one of which is under construction).
Staff to resident ratio	1:6 from 7:00 a.m. to 3:00 p.m.; 1:6 from 3:00 p.m. to 11:00 p.m.; 1:12 from 11:00 p.m. to 7:00 a.m.
Site/context	Suburban, residential area, near shopping and other commercial facilities.
Size	6,000 square feet (approximate)
Date of completion	October 1990
Architects	Erlick, Gunson & Associates, Inc., Port Washington, Wisconsin

Figure 2.20   Plan of New Perspective Group Home #4, Mequon, Wisconsin.

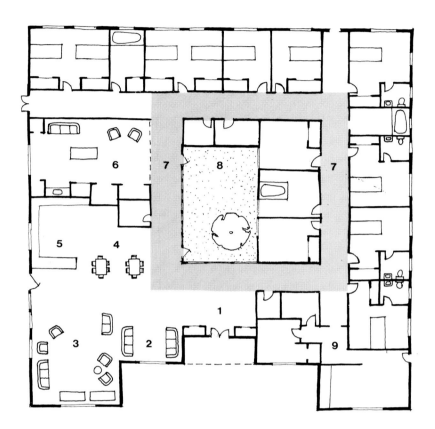

1   entry
2   lounge
3   living/activity room
4   dining room
5   domestic kitchen
6   enclosable activity room
7   wandering path
8   central courtyard
9   auxiliary apartment

Noninstitutional Image

+ This is a house-size building with typical residential features—single story, pitched roof, and a side yard.

+ The auxiliary apartment (*9*) adds to the residential image both in terms of house form and programmatically. The resident caregiver keeps the unit's pet and maintains a permanent presence.

Positive Outdoor Space

+ The central outdoor courtyard (*8*) is a primary organizing feature of the plan. In addition to providing a secure outdoor activity space with a protected micro-climate, it provides daylight and windows to five internal rooms and the main public area. It also reduces the "corridor" portion of the wandering path.

Wandering Path

+ The path (*7*) around the core is partially a conventional corridor. However, more than half of the path overlooks activity (*6*), dining (*4*), and living (*3*) areas.

– The emergency doors at the corridors' ends are a tempting target for wandering residents, who may attempt to travel outdoors to the enclosed yard.

Entry and Transition

– The entry area is too close and too exposed to the main activity area. This may result in disruptive behavior during visitors' coming and going.

Variety of Activity Areas

+ The small unit has a variety of activity spaces: the small lounge (*2*), the more public living room (*3*), the dining room (*4*), and the kitchen (*5*) are loci of activity; the multipurpose activity room (*6*) can be a secure, quiet room for one or two residents away from the rest of the group.

Background
History and development

The owners of New Perspective first entered the business of residential health care provision with a renovation of a single-family house for eight residents. The firm has since built four group homes in the Milwaukee metropolitan area, with the fifth home presently under construction.

As the number of New Perspective group homes increased, their management simultaneously standardized and professionalized: a board of directors was established, management structure within and between the homes became better defined, and policies of operation became more explicit (see under "The Staff").

Group Home #4 is the most recently completed of the New Perspective homes, occupied since the winter of 1991. (Already, however, Group Home #5 is entering the final stages of construction, situated on the same lot as #4, separated by a back yard that both homes will eventually share.) Advertisement was not necessary to fill Group Home #4; the company and its owner have developed a reputation in the community based on the success of earlier homes. This reputation prompted numerous referrals. In fact, all residents learned of the home through word of mouth or recommendation by others in the community.

Construction costs

Construction costs for the home totaled approximately $600,000, although this was uncharacteristicly inexpensive because of the low cost paid for the site.

Cost for care

Residents pay between $65 and $76 a day, with private rooms and baths the most expensive (and popular) option and shared rooms with a bathroom in the corridor the least.

Services

New Perspective employees arrange services, such as transportation to physicians and beauty parlor services, on a fee-per-service basis for residents.

Organizational and Social Environment
The staff

Staff members at Group Home #4 include a manager, an assistant manager, and aides, in addition to an activity coordinator and a massage therapist who operate among all four homes. Staffing includes two staff members on the first and second shifts and one on the third shift. Light housekeeping duties are assigned to each shift, with a weekly cleaning service managing all major cleaning. Recent changes have been implemented with the intention of increasing staff members' professionalism. These include professional screening and testing of each applicant, increases in staff salaries, and the use of time clocks.

The residents

Nine of the eleven residents of Group Home #4 are women. (At the time of our visit, one resident had recently been relocated. A new resident was expected to move in within the week.) Residents vary in the stage of their dementia—from those in the early stages of the disease who remain fairly cognitively intact to nonverbal residents in advanced stages. All residents are mobile, either independently or with the assistance of a walker. Incontinence has proven to be more common among the residents than expected (based on the literature and on family and resident self-reports); most residents are at least occasionally bladder-incontinent, although the facility does not accept residents who are regularly bowel-incontinent.

The families

Most residents come from the local community, where either they or a family member have resided. Visiting is a prevalent activity in the home; family members come and go both informally and frequently. Visitors are encouraged to arrive unannounced and to join in activities and meals at any time (although visiting after 9:30 or 10:00 p.m. is discouraged). Visitors have become well acquainted with many of the residents, reinforcing the description of the home and its residents as an "extended family." They frequently take residents out for day trips and even short vacations.

Program Description

Three structured activities are scheduled each day: the first after breakfast, the second in the afternoon, and a third quiet activity in the evening. An activity director was recently hired to coordinate activities, gather supplies, and instruct staff members on activities for all four New Perspective homes. Music-based activities, such as sing-a-longs and weekly dances, are especially popular. Occasionally, activities are brought to the home, such as visiting babies from a local child care center. Residents are also taken to outside activities on occasion, most frequently during summer months. These trips have included visits to the senior citizen center and an evening cruise on a river boat. "Bumper bowling" at the nearby bowling alley is also popular. In this version, large inflatable tubes are placed in the gutters, acting as bumpers to guide the ball down the alley to the pins. All players knock down pins every turn. This strategy does not deter from the challenge of the sport for those residents who are more physically capable and yet allows all residents to feel positive about participation in the activity.

Physical Environment
Entry area

Upon entering the home, one steps into what resembles (as it is, in fact) a residential entry area in a large, open-plan home. Visitors must ring to be admitted, as the front door is monitored by a loud, potentially disruptive security alarm. The major public spaces of the home are visible and the layout is comprehensible immediately upon entering. Two wicker chairs next to the door form a small seating alcove.

Outdoor spaces

Across from the activity room is the interior, central courtyard. Windows along two walls admit light into the home from this space and allow additional (albeit rather unexciting) views to the outdoors. The courtyard can be used in the spring and summer for breakfast outside and as an additional activity area. The owner recounts how, in the winter, staff members in another New Perspective home lined residents up along the hallway and devised an afternoon's entertainment by building a snowman in the courtyard and throwing snowballs at the windows. Although there was no furniture in the courtyard during the case study visit (in February), a patio table and chairs had been purchased for use in warmer months.

The backyard connects Group Home #4 to Group Home #5, under construction in the adjacent lot. When it is landscaped, the backyard will be a common outdoor space shared by residents of both facilities.

Wandering path

Group Home #4 is designed around the concept of a circular wandering path, which provides the residents with a continuous loop for wandering devoid of most frustrating dead ends that would force residents to stop and turn back. In this home, the wandering path dictated a donut-shaped plan wrapped around a central interior courtyard. Most residents walk around the facility on their own, without a need for constant staff supervision. The staff to resident ratio permits staff members to know each resident well and to judge when residents may have become "lost" or disoriented and which residents require supervision while wandering. A television monitoring system in the corridor was once considered to ensure adequate supervision of wandering residents; however, this solution was perceived as institutional and detrimental to the residential nature and goals of the home. Instead, staff members walk with those residents who require supervision.

Living rooms and social spaces

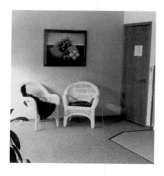

Figure 2.21
The domestic nature and arrangement of furnishings contribute to the noninstitutional ambience of the facility.

Public spaces are arranged in an open great-room plan reminiscent of traditional Southern houses, with living room, den, kitchen, and dining room flowing into each other in a relaxed and informal manner. This scheme was intended to provide heightened visibility between the spaces, enhancing the caregivers' ability to survey most of the residents simultaneously. The home is decorated in a country style in soft shades of blue and mauve, selected to be soothing and restful (fig. 2.21).

The living area is divided into a large and a small space by a half-wall partition; the smaller of the two spaces includes two facing sofas and is used as a quiet area. The main living area contains a TV, a radio, and each resident's individual armchair. Residents are encouraged to bring their own chair from home, but one is provided for any resident who does not. This area is carpeted (as is most of the facility, with the exception of the kitchen area, enclosable activity room, and bathrooms). There is an absence of strong odors in the home, including both cleaning solvents and urine, possibly due at least in part to the newness of the facility. Every opportunity to admit sunlight and views to the outdoors has been realized, giving the home a warm, sunny feeling. A ceiling fan in the living room keeps the home at a warm but comfortable temperature. In one corner of the living area sits a canary in a bird cage, one resident's pet that accompanied her to the home.

Kitchen/dining area

The kitchen is distinguished from the great room by a change from carpet to linoleum and by the location of a kitchen island, which serves as an informal observation post for surveying residents in the living area (fig. 2.22). In former New Perspective homes, kitchen cabinets had been built above the island,

Figure 2.22
Overview of the kitchen and dining area. This space is a locus for household-related activities, as well as an excellent vantage point for unobtrusive surveillance of the entrance, great room, interior courtyard, and parts of the wandering path.

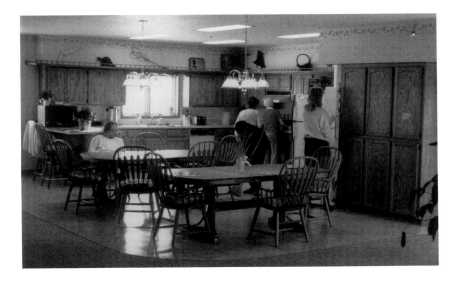

creating a full-wall partition. However, this reduced visibility into the living room; at employees' suggestion, a simple island was substituted in Group Home #4.

Since all food for the home is cooked on the premises, there was a need to optimize storage space in the kitchen. Kitchen walls are lined with full-wall oak cupboards for food and dish storage. Cupboards that contain dangerous equipment or utensils are lockable; however, most are left open to encourage residents to make a cup of tea for themselves or to participate in kitchen activities when they choose. Two rectangular tables for six are used for meals and some activities. (Messy activities such as painting take place at the plastic table in the activity room.) During the case study visit, two residents and an aide prepared egg salad together for a group meal.

Activity spaces

Adjacent to the kitchen is a large activity room used for group activities, dances, and the weekly "beauty shop" during the beautician's visit. Situated in one corner is a convertible beautician's sink that can be opened when needed and that resembles a regular bureau when not in use. A washer and dryer occupy one of the large closets. A second closet contains games used during visits with family members (including toys for visiting children, such as the child-sized basketball hoop in one corner of the room). The third, locked closet holds residents' medications.

The activity room receives sunlight from two large windows into the backyard and from the open indoor courtyard across the hall. It is defined both by a change in floor surface—from carpet to linoleum—and by a simple wooden "fence" with a dutch door. This was installed to accommodate one resident who wandered constantly and rummaged through her own and others' possessions when not supervised. Because she had put small objects into her mouth on several occasions, staff members were afraid to leave the resident unobserved and yet had insufficient resources for constant supervision. The design of the activity room was devised as an alternative to allow the resident to remain in the home. After consulting with her family members, the fence and gate (with a child-proof latch that the resident cannot open) were added to the activity room. Now, when necessary, the resident is left alone in the activity room and given plenty of safe objects through which to sort and rummage. Staff members report that she enjoys this arrangement and does not feel isolated because she can hear activity in the great room and is not completely separated in a fully enclosed room.

The activity room often functions as a place for family celebrations or birthday parties for residents and their family members. In addition, it houses a small desk used by staff members for paperwork.

Residents' rooms

Residents' rooms line two sides of the square plan. Residents choose between three room options: two rooms are shared, four are private, and four are private rooms with a personal bathroom. Prices vary from $23,000 to $27,000 a year accordingly.

Each resident's room has a unique wallpaper pattern and a different color bedcover and curtains, all complementing the blue and mauve color scheme. Materials were selected to be soothing and reminiscent of those styles likely to be found in residents' former homes. Each resident has his or her own closet and dresser. Beds and dressers are provided by the home, and all residents are encouraged to decorate their rooms with personal items and furnishings from home. Family members have taken advantage of this opportunity by helping residents to decorate their rooms according to personal preferences. Each resident room is wired for TV, cable television, and private phone lines, which residents may install if they choose. Staff members report that this option is sometimes appropriate for residents who are more cognitively intact and who occasionally may watch TV in their own room when they desire privacy or may appreciate the opportunity to keep in touch with family members and friends over the phone. Most residents' telephones are programmed for a few frequently called numbers, relieving the resident of the need to remember phone numbers. In one ingenious solution, the family of a resident who made frequent long distance calls throughout the night provided her with a telephone with a timer device, rendering the phone inoperational during nighttime hours.

Resident rooms are equipped with emergency call buttons for use by staff members to request additional help, particularly during the third shift, when only one aide is on duty. The call buttons signal to the kitchen and to an attached auxiliary apartment. Although the call buttons were not intended for resident use, they are occasionally mistaken by residents for light switches and signaled inadvertently, prompting the owner to suggest that, in future homes, call buttons will be placed in less conspicuous locations in resident rooms.

Outside residents' rooms, construction paper signs identify each room with the resident's name. Some family members have also installed more permanent, "dignified" (yet ironically more institutional) name signs, of the type common in offices. Staff members indicate that residents would be unable to identify their rooms without the signs (despite the rooms' variety in color and decor, adopted for personalization rather than identification) and that some cannot identify their rooms without assistance even with the signs. Doors to some residents' rooms are kept shut to discourage those residents prone to rummaging. Staff members encourage respect for residents' privacy by knocking before entering rooms.

Toilet and shower/ tub rooms

Most of the common bathrooms are interspersed between the residents' rooms. One exception, a powder room, is located near the public spaces, between the kitchen and activity room. All bathrooms are equipped for use by handicapped people. Staff members have found that all residents function better when provided with extra room to maneuver and that grab bars installed for support during transferring help to reassure all residents when using the toilet, as many are afraid to lower themselves onto the toilet seat without support (because of common dementia-related problems in depth perception). The powder room door had been installed to open toward the kitchen, allowing residents to see and locate the bathroom easily. However, at the request of the residents, who disapproved of the view into the bathroom from the kitchen table, the door was rehinged to open toward the activity room.

Three additional common bathrooms are distributed throughout the facility. The first of these includes a walk-in, wheel-in shower, the most popular bathing option for residents. The shower's gently sloping floor allows water to flow into two floor drains. (Past experience had demonstrated that one drain was insufficient to remove all water.) This arrangement allows residents to be showered in a wheelchair if necessary. A heat lamp and auxiliary heater were installed to maintain a comfortable bathroom temperature during bathing. Reinforced grab bars were substituted for ordinary towel racks, as residents also use towel racks for support. The owner suggested that the choice of colors in the bathroom (standard institutional beige) and the lack of decoration contribute to the somewhat institutional appearance of this space.

An additional, smaller bathroom includes a residential bathtub, used less often for bathing (perhaps because of the necessity of stepping over its deep side to enter). A third, large bathroom contains a whirlpool very popular among residents. (This also requires residents to negotiate the depth of the tub to enter. Entering is normally accomplished in stages: sitting residents on the edge, swinging their feet around, and lowering them into the tub.) During the case study visit, the massage therapist was giving weekly massages in this room, another activity residents enjoy.

Some residents at Group Home #4 have regular problems with incontinence; because this symptom can occur quite early in the disease, the owner regularly accepts bladder-incontinent residents who are otherwise able to function in the home. Diapering and toileting schedules are both used to combat this problem. One resident had particular trouble locating the bathroom due to a habit of walking with her head down, usually right past the bathroom.

Staff members added a rubber mat with the large word TOILET outside the bathroom door to attract her attention. (They are still uncertain whether this strategy has had any effect.)

Absence of staff "retreat"/lounge areas

Staff members in Group Home #4 are encouraged to interact with the residents as much as possible, in keeping with the noninstitutional, homelike care philosophy of the facility. In support of this philosophy, staff members complete all paperwork at a small, unobtrusive staff desk in the corner of the activity room rather than at a designated staff work space or room. Although staff members have complained that the location of this desk in the activity room dictates that all paperwork be locked in the drawers away from residents, the owner is satisfied that this arrangement minimizes the amount of time spent on paperwork and the amount of space dedicated to this activity.

Group Home #4 is attached to an auxiliary staff apartment, which opens into the facility along the resident room corridor. The apartment also has a separate entrance. The interior connection to the group home allows the staff member living in the apartment to enter the facility quickly if necessary. In an additional convenience, this staff apartment also serves as the home of the facility's dog. The dog is a pet of the staff member living in the apartment and accompanies her to the home during her shifts. This arrangement dispels ambiguity concerning responsibility for the dog and provides flexibility, as the dog is left in the apartment when residents are agitated or engaged in activities demanding concentration (both potential sources of conflict in group homes with pets).

Equipment and furnishings

Group Home #4 has quality finishes, surfaces, and furnishings, such as the oak trim, cabinets, and furnishings in the kitchen; the high-quality bathroom fixtures; and similar touches throughout the home. Additional notable features include the electrical outlets placed in the floor to prevent residents from tripping over cords and the rounded oak handrails that surround the hallway wandering path.

Pathways Project

Address	Pembroke Pines Broward County, FL
Owner	Miami Jewish Home and Hospital for the Aged (MJHHA) 151 Northeast 52nd Street Miami, FL 33137 (305) 751-8626
Staff contact	Judith K. Williams, Ph.D., Director of Policy and Planning, MJHHA
Facility type	Self-contained continuum of care campus for people with dementia and their caregivers
Residents	Residents will span all stages of the disease, from late stage 1 through late stage 3. Caregivers will also reside on the campus, both with residents and alone.
Site/context	A site of 25 acres in a typical, suburban, low-rise and single-family residential area
Size	25 acres (approximate)
Date of completion	The Pathways community will be developed and occupied in three distinct phases, the first of which is planned for 1993.
Architects	KJA Architects, Somerville, Massachusetts

Information about this case study was derived primarily from MJHHA program and design documents; all drawings are by KJA Architects.

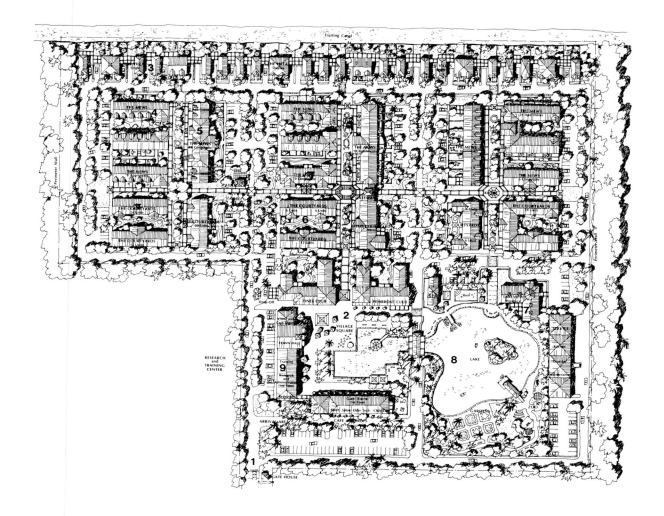

1   entry

2   village square

3   single family houses or duplexes

4   row houses

5   assisted living units

6   comprehensive care

7   hospice

8   lake

9   administrative/research area

The following items were distilled from jury comments pertaining to the winning entry in an invited competition to design the master plan for Pathways.

+ The plan offers a noninstitutional, natural image by conforming to conventions of residential developments in Florida.

+ The mews provide an opportunity for social activity, interaction, and secure wandering.

+ Cooperative care-giving units provide a connection to the services of the village while allowing care-giving spouses to maintain their autonomy.

+ Wandering and circulation are controlled at a number of different scales: the unit, the garden, the courtyard, and the mews. This provides a secure wandering environment, with increasing levels of challenge and distance from home.

+ The various building types are designed to meet dementia-specific needs and problems.

− Critical comments centered on several design and locational features, including

• the need for greater hierarchy to the mews, making some more dominant than others

• the need to decentralize some activities from the town square to other zones

• the need to remove road and pedestrian movement conflicts.

Background
History

Pathways, a residential and service community for clients with Alzheimer's disease and their caregivers, is being developed by the Miami Jewish Home and Hospital for the Aged at Douglas Gardens in a public/private partnership with the state of Florida. The goal is to develop a supportive residential environment to keep people with dementia and their caregivers active and together longer. In 1988, Florida legislation, through the Department of Health and Rehabilitative Services (HRS) appropriated planning funds to MJHHA for Pathways, with the intent of leasing state land to the project. Since that time, MJHHA has worked with HRS on the Pathways program development plan and various site assessment and capacity reports. The Pathways sublease for twenty-five acres of land in southwest Broward County was approved by the governor and cabinet in January 1990.

The architectural master site plan for Pathways is the result of a design competition in which three firms were invited to submit their proposed schemes for use of the site. Review of the three proposals was based on criteria that incorporate basic elements of the Pathways' guiding principles. The architect selected to provide the final master plan was Barry Korobkin of KJA Architects, Somerville, Massachusetts.

Development process

The program for Pathways was developed through a planning process that included an extensive literature review, work with the state of Florida, and consultation throughout the process with recognized experts in the care of people with dementia and the design of facilities specifically for people with dementia. An initial result of the process was a set of guiding principles and therapeutic goals (discussed above) that directed subsequent program and architectural design.

Goals
Key therapeutic goals

- *Permit both independence and control.* Pathways planning and design are geared toward the delivery of the least restrictive environment possible. Adequate, safe outdoor and indoor spaces permit free wandering. Ready access to the outside is deemed important, as are relatively short walking distances for daily activities. In addition, residents' normal life patterns will be maintained through the use of both design and programming.
- *Ensure accessibility for mobility impaired residents and caregivers.* All buildings will be entered directly from grade, and all second floor space will be serviced by elevators.
- *Provide a noninstitutional setting.* To realize the goal of maintaining a homelike environment, design was planned at a small scale, with people with dementia living in small "family" units and sharing small-scale social spaces.
- *Offer a broad spectrum of services.* This goal is intended to ensure that the community meets the individual needs of caregivers and people with dementia throughout the disease. Services provided will include assessment and care planning, care coordination, specialized health services, education

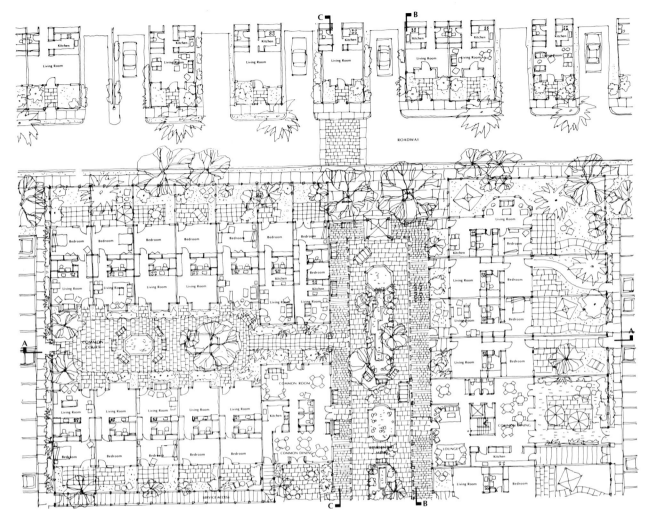

Figure 2.24

A typical pedestrian mews. (Drawing by KJA Architects.)

and training, day and respite care, caregiver training and support, home care, environmental adaptation, and social activities. The range of residential options and support facilities provided also support this goal.

- *Accommodate individual differences.* Pathways will adapt to a range of impairments in both people with dementia and their caregivers. Additionally, various living environments will be accommodated in the Pathways community.
- *Provide stimulation and challenge.* Realization of this goal translates into the provision of social spaces of varying types, both outside and inside. The plan is for a social atmosphere, rather than a medical or nursing atmosphere. Finally, adequate space for activities for all residents is integral to the design.
- *Maintain good security.* Security in outdoor and indoor spaces has two foci: external, concerned with protecting residents from intruders or other

threats from the outside, and internal, concerned with such matters as medical emergencies and lost wanderers.

Family support goals

- *Focus on the family caregivers.* The needs of family caregivers comprise a significant source of direction for the planning and design of the Pathways campus. This is true for caregivers living with and without their family member with dementia, throughout all stages of the disease.

Research, education, and application goals

- *Promote and support research, evaluation, and training.* These activities are a primary component of the Pathways program. Research will emphasize service interventions, desirable characteristics of living environments, and effects of services and environments on caregivers and people with dementia. Training will be provided to caregivers, both professional and informal, and to people with dementia. The building environment of Pathways is being designed to facilitate research and training.

- *Support replication of parts of the community to other sites.* The ability to replicate indicates that universal design principles are applied, construction and the program are affordable, the model is adaptable to other sites, spaces are flexible, and individual components can be changed in response to evaluation and market forces.

Physical Environment
Description of the plan

Pathways planners anticipate gradual resident occupancy and are conducting financial planning and design and development accordingly. Phase 1 densities and design are intended to allow the complex to be self-sustaining if subsequent phases are not built.

Principles of spatial arrangement

The Pathways site is divided into five blocks by a *grid of village roads,* providing full car and truck access to all development on the site and easements for all utilities. In this way, the community is organized by its pedestrian and vehicular circulation requirements.

Figure 2.25 (*left*)
Village Center arrival area.
(Drawing by KJA Architects.)

Figure 2.26 (*right*)
Assisted living courtyard apartments. (Drawing by KJA Architects.)

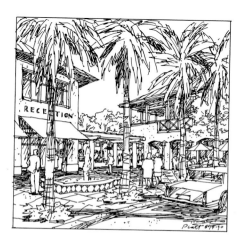
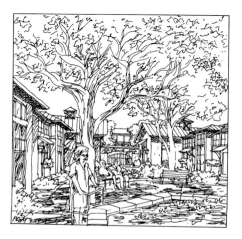

A *pedestrian mews* is sited in the center of each residential block, providing a street focus for residential neighborhoods leading to the village square (fig. 2.24).

The *village square* at the center of the campus serves as a focal point for all surrounding buildings (fig. 2.25).

Housing options

Residential units will be planned in three distinct neighborhoods, each with single-family or duplex houses, row houses, and courtyard houses. Neighborhoods will be developed in distinct phases.

Assisted living units will be housed in two types of arrangements: apartments grouped around shared living and dining spaces, where access to apartments is independent of involvement in shared spaces, and congregate houses, where apartments are organized within larger buildings including living, dining, and recreation areas. A number of options will be provided: courtyard houses (fig. 2.26), row and congregate houses, gallery access units, and second story apartments.

Comprehensive care will be provided in the following options: twenty-four-resident unit houses, divided into subclusters for six and twelve residents; a 12-unit house; and a 6-unit group home. All units will be designed with lockable kitchenettes and private bathrooms. Most rooms would be private, but shared rooms would also be included.

Villas are also planned as single-family detached and side-by-side duplex single-story houses (fig. 2.27). These are designed for both caregiver privacy and support by proximity to other units and services. Cooperative housing would abut quality market-rate housing on the adjoining parcel.

A *hospice* will be constructed outside the immediate residential neighborhoods, as it requires little involvement with the rest of the facility. A single, twenty-unit, two-story house near the lake is provided.

Figure 2.27 (*left*)
The villas—caregiver cooperative homes. (Drawing by KJA Architects.)

Figure 2.28 (*right*)
View from the center's Inn over the lake area. (Drawing by KJA Architects.)

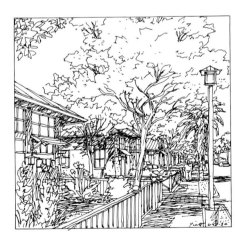
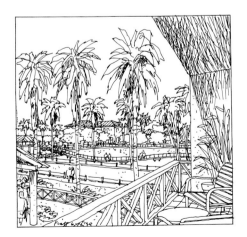

Outdoor spaces　　　　The village square at the center of the campus serves as a reception area for people from the outside; as the center for research and administration, training, and conferences; and as the commercial, recreational, and "work" destination for residents. Outdoor, fenced courtyards and yards and covered pedestrian ways connect all buildings.

　　　A required drainage lake, fenced securely, will provide an attractive amenity for the campus (fig. 2.28). The lake will be surrounded by walking paths. Its planned location is near a swimming pool and sauna and the hospice.

Saint Ann Day Care Center

Address	3221 South Lake Drive St. Francis, WI 53207 (414) 744-1160 (414) 482-1340
Owner	Independent Living Services, Order of Sisters of St. Francis of Assisi
Staff contact	Sister Edna Lonergan, Executive Director, St. Ann Adult Day Care
Facility type	Dementia day care center. A separate adult day care center for persons with physical disabilities is also located on the premises.
Participants	Anticipated total of 20, with 17 participants on a typical day
Staff	Three full-time staff, as well as an occupational therapist, activity programmer, gerontologist, and music therapist shared with the other adult day care unit
Staffing ratio	Approximately 1:4
Site/context	The center is housed in a renovated former kitchen in a basement area within the convent campus. The campus is located in a residential area in a small community south of Milwaukee.
Size (approximate)	Main room: 784 square feet Service area: 350 square feet Administration: 100 square feet
Date of completion	November 1987 (walkway completed in the spring of 1989)
Architects	C.G. Schmidt, Contractor, ELO Interiors
Publication	Lonergan, E. (1986). Holistic model of day care. Unpublished monograph. Cardinal Strich College, Milwaukee.

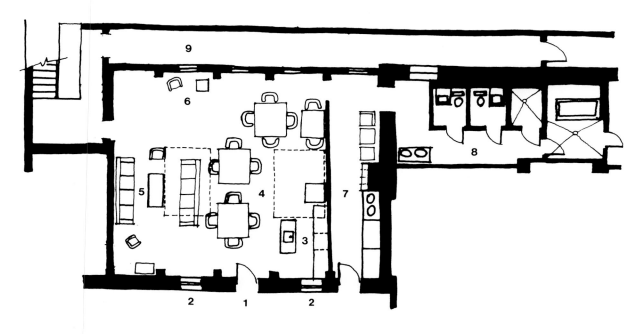

1   entrance
2   observation windows
3   kitchen area
4   dining/activities area
5   living/small group area
6   multipurpose area
7   laundry
8   toilet and bathrooms
9   sun room/pacing area

Noninstitutional Image

+ The unit is a good example of a utility area renovation in a windowless basement space, turned into a domestic and residential great room. The size and scale of the room are just right for the group of about twenty and yet are within the range of regular living and dining rooms in a house. The interior finishes and furniture also radiate the atmosphere of "home." Even the fact that this is a windowless space does not affect the interior adversely: the skylights and the light from the skylit pacing area provide daylight and a sense of orientation to the outdoors.

Wandering

− The pacing area along the external side of the great room (9) is a long corridor, skylit with frosted glass. Because of its narrow width and dead end, it does not provide opportunities for continuous wandering, nor does it offer activities or meaningful destinations.

Domestic Kitchen and Intimate Dining

+ The residential kitchen (3) with an island table, the adjoining dining area (4) with four tables, and the seating area with sofas and stuffed chairs support an activity program that is based on familiar daily activities. Both the program and the physical environment contribute further to a noninstitutional environment. The kitchen is the locus of activity in the unit, and it serves as a point for unobtrusive surveillance by the staff.

Entry and Transition

+ The entry hall (1) is buffered from the great room by a door and one-way windows, which allow unobtrusive observation into the room by visitors and relatives. The separation of "coming and going" activity from the residents reduces the potential for disruption and agitation so often associated with entryways.

Background

History

In January 1983, recognizing the special problems of the old-old and their need for a support system to prevent premature institutionalization, the Sisters of St. Francis of Assisi opened the St. Ann Day Care Program. It became evident within a short time that day care clients with Alzheimer's disease or related dementias required an adapted environment. The unique needs of the memory-impaired client dictated an environment that was stimulating but not distracting, one that was simple and less confusing than the ordinary day care setting.

After this realization, money was raised to renovate a suite of rooms to provide the adapted environment for a new day care program for people with AD, which has been in operation since November 1987, providing day care and opportunities for socialization for participants, respite for caregivers, and education and training for community and family members.

Mission

The mission of the St. Ann Adult Day Center has been twofold: to improve the quality of life for individuals who are struggling to remain at home and to give support to their caregivers. Efforts are made to maintain an atmosphere of friendship, prayer, faith sharing, and hospitality among staff members and participants.

Costs

Participants pay $29.50 per day. Moderate financial aid is available.

Services

Day care services are available Monday through Friday from 8:00 a.m. to 4:00 p.m. (until 5:30 p.m. on Tuesdays) and on Saturdays from 8:00 a.m. to 3:30 p.m. Bathing and grooming services are also available for an additional charge.

Goals

Key therapeutic goals

- *Focus on emotions.* Given that the emotional awareness of people with dementia remains despite cognitive losses, the staff emphasizes affective communication.
- *Provide moderated levels of stimulation.*

Organizational and Social Environment

The staff

There are three full-time staff members in the day care center, as well as an occupational therapist and a music therapist shared with another program of adult day care. A staff to client ratio of approximately 1:4 is maintained throughout the day.

The participants

Participants are accepted until the final stages of the disease, as long as they are not disruptive to the program. Most participants enter the program during stage 2, and some come to the program from the affiliated integrated day care center.

The families

The center provides participant and family education and support groups for caregivers.

Program Description

The St. Ann Center's model of care is not a "medical" or "social service" one, but is rather a holistic model based on love and acceptance. The program focuses on familiar daily activities and is as functional and simple as possible. Group activities are provided throughout the day, with a quicker pace of more challenging activities maintained in the morning (most participants' attention spans shorten as the day progresses). There is an effort to introduce small children and age peers (retired nuns) into the center. Hug therapy—with stuffed animals and other participants—is felt to be very important. Therapeutic exercises, training in activities of daily living, and leisure time activities and outings are equally represented in the activity program.

Although the goal is one of sustained group activities, the staff provides as much individual attention as required.

Figure 2.30
Four activity areas—kitchen, dining room, living room (*shown at right*), and multipurpose space—are distinguished within one large space.

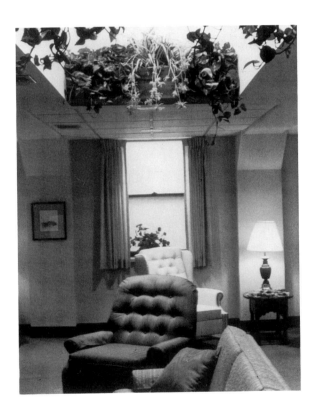

Physical Environment
Description of the plan

There are four activity areas (kitchen, dining room, living room, and multipurpose space) within one larger space (fig. 2.30). The areas are defined by furnishings and skylights, with a service area located behind a screen wall. There is a walkway for wandering in a former open area, now enclosed with a skylight added overhead.

Entry area

The St. Ann Day Care Center is located in the basement of a convent. The entrance "hall" is primarily intended for visitors—it is not envisioned or used as an activity area for participants. The hall is furnished with solid, heavy, non-institutional furnishings and is designed to be calming and quiet, to minimize overstimulation during coming and going. One-way windows into the center allow unobtrusive observation by visitors, architects, and students, without disturbing the participants.

Great room

The main activity spaces of the center compose a "great room," including a living room, dining area, multipurpose area, and kitchenette. Skylights—filled with nontoxic plants—admit natural light into the living area. Other plants in the room are artificial, so that participants do not eat them. Sofas and over-stuffed chairs are grouped into two small, primary arrangements to accommodate small group and private conversations. All furnishings, wall hangings, and materials and surfaces are elegant and homelike, in soft, muted, calming pastel colors (fig. 2.31).

Figure 2.31
The residential nature and arrangement of furnishings, along with special touches such as afghans, skylighting, and plants, enhance the homelike atmosphere of this renovated-basement day care center.

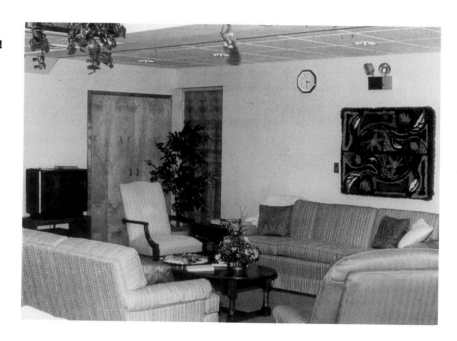

Kitchen/dining areas

The kitchenette fills one wall of the living area. Complete with stove (with cover), microwave oven (both controlled by wall switches), refrigerator, and a work island with a sink for doing dishes, this area was intended (and functions) as a node of activity in the center. Tables are square—making it easier for residents to set the table for meals—with rounded corners (fig. 2.32).

Wandering path

Behind the living room is a newly constructed, enclosed wandering hall, temperature controlled for year-round use. The wandering path is lit from above by frosted glass skylights to control glare; it is safe and accessible for independent use.

Figure 2.32
The kitchen island serves as a locus of activity for participants—dish washing and drying, food preparation—and a point for unobtrusive surveillance of the great room by staff members.

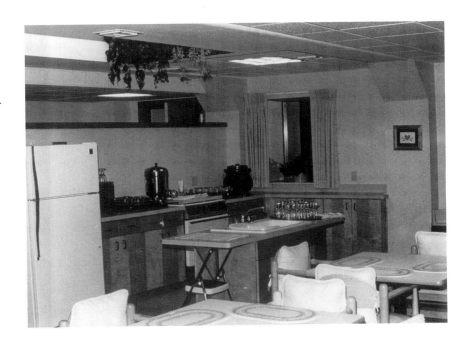

Toilet and shower/ tub rooms

The bathroom area is color coded in teal from the living room, cueing residents to follow these colors to reach the toilets. International symbol signs to the toilets are visible from the living room. Inside, a grooming area with a mirror and shelf used for beauty and grooming activities is located adjacent to two toilet rooms (handicapped accessible). A walk-in shower room with a sloping floor can be used for bathing participants while seated. Beyond this, a small space houses a whirlpool Apollo tub, accessible on three sides for ease in assisting participants.

Laundry area

Behind the kitchen, out of view and "earshot" of residents, is the laundry area, complete with a clothes washer and dryer and a dishwasher. These appliances are located where the noise and activity they generate will not be irritating to participants. In addition, because dishes washed by hand by participants must be "rewashed" in the dishwasher for health and safety reasons, the dishwasher is located out of sight to avoid offending or distracting participants.

Staff "retreat" or lounge areas

A small room in the entrance hall is used as a student classroom and conference area. It is furnished with a desk and space for paperwork and a rocking chair and stuffed animal. (The space serves a secondary function as a quiet room for agitated residents.) The adjoining handicapped-accessible "guest" bathroom is used by staff and visitors.

Equipment and furnishings

Furnishings and equipment are intended to satisfy a number of criteria. First, windows have frosted glass to eliminate glare. All furnishings are of a residential design. Chairs are sturdy and stable, with extra padding to assist clients in raising themselves, and a clear contrast is maintained between furniture and floors (as well as between each chair/armrest).

Traditional, recognizable kitchen faucets were selected to be familiar to and usable by residents. In particular, bathroom faucets were selected to be easy to manipulate. Specially weighted and textured silverware is intended to be easy for participants to "feel," and plates and placemats were selected for high contrast with the table and are easy to see while eating.

Materials and surfaces

Materials and surfaces have likewise been carefully selected. There is carpeting in all "living" areas and tile in service areas. Walls, tiles, and laminates are all matte finished, and finely textured wallpaper was selected. All living room furnishings have a residential finish in fabric heavily coated with a spray-on fabric protector. In addition, color codes and pictograms are used to identify bathrooms.

Therapeutic Garden, Sunset Haven Home for the Aged

Address	163 First Avenue Welland, Ontario L3C 9Y5, Canada (416) 735-1620
Owner	Regional Niagara Senior Citizens Department
Staff contact	Peter Papp, Administrator
Facility type	Skilled nursing facility
Residents	348 residents at various levels of functioning
Staff	The therapeutic garden is open to residents at all times, with and without staff supervision. However, staff members, relatives, and volunteers often accompany residents in the garden.
Staff to resident ratio	Varies depending on specific activity in the garden
Site/context	The garden is situated between—and enclosed by—two wings of the home, on a rectangular site. It can be entered from the building at its two ends.
Size	30,000-square-foot garden
Date of completion	Garden constructed in 1979
Architects	Conceptualized by Douglas H. Rapelje, Lawrence Crawford, and Peter Papp. Design by Vertechs, Toronto.
Publications	Rapelje, D.H., and Crawford, L. (1987). Creating lively park-spaces for mentally frail seniors in long term care. *Recreation Canada,* December, pp.23–27. Lovering, M.J. (1990). Alzheimer's disease and outdoor space: Issues in environmental design. *American Journal of Alzheimer's Care and Related Disorders and Research,* May/June, pp. 33–40. Rapelje, D.G., Papp, P.P., and Crawford, L. (1981). Creating a therapeutic park for the mentally frail. *Dimensions in Health Service,* September, pp. 12–14.

Figure 2.33   Plan of the therapeutic garden at Sunset Haven Home for the Aged, Welland, Ontario, Canada.

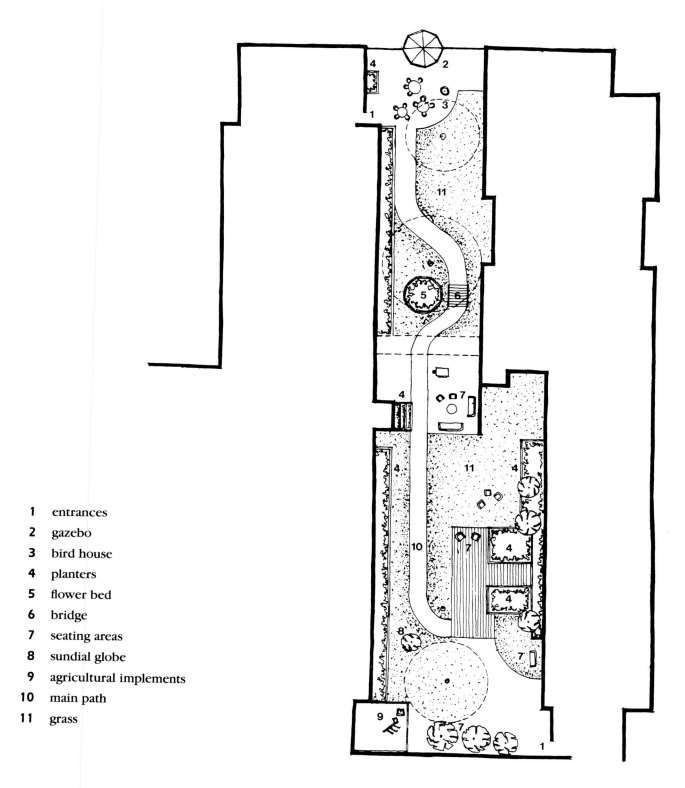

1   entrances
2   gazebo
3   bird house
4   planters
5   flower bed
6   bridge
7   seating areas
8   sundial globe
9   agricultural implements
10 main path
11 grass

Range of Activity Spaces

+ The extensive park—30,000 square feet—includes a rich variety of activity spaces, places, and objects. The grounds include sunny and shaded zones, with several large trees, grassy areas, and a continuous concrete path. Planters and small plazas offer a variety of seating arrangements, from built-in benches to regular chairs. The gazebo (2), bird house (3), flower bed (5), and agricultural implements (9) provide varied stimulation, degrees of privacy, and different exposures to sun and wind.

Entry and Transition

− A major shortcoming of the park is its restricted physical and visual access: the two entry/exit points (1) are situated in remote areas of the facility that are difficult to find and identify. The park is also visually obscured from the public spaces in the building. Built as an addition, the park is not integrated in any meaningful way with the building's interiors.

Things from the Past

+ Familiar objects such as the country water pump and several agricultural implements (9) are useful catalysts for reminiscence and social integration.

− More abstract and "out of context" objects such as the oversized sundial (8) are not recognizable by residents and add visual clutter.

Sensory Stimulation without Stress

+ The overall sensory effect of the park is positive. The park provides opportunities for variations in levels of stimulation, from passive bird watching to wandering or participating in programmed activities.

− Earlier experiments introduced running water and a bridge over the stream (6). This proved to be stressful and disorienting for residents.

Background
History

In 1978, after the publication of research findings regarding the influence of the physical environment on the experience and behavior of residents of special care units, administrators of the Senior Citizens Department of the Regional Municipality of Niagara decided to pursue the design of an outdoor park for mentally impaired and confused residents.

The development process: staff involvement in planning and construction

The park was designed and constructed over a twelve-month period. Staff members were consulted by the landscape architect. Most construction was completed by the facility's own maintenance staff. The participation in planning and construction was related to a high level of excitement and commitment to the garden by all those involved.

Mission

The mission of the park was to provide an alternative activity area, with new and different sources of physical and mental stimulation.

Funding

Funds for the garden came from the Regional Niagara Senior Citizens Department, as well as from special fund-raising campaigns.

Goals
Key therapeutic goals

- Reduce confinement and the use of restraints.
- Provide opportunities for activity and free mobility.
- Ensure safety.
- Provide physical and mental stimulation.

Physical Environment
Plan description
Park features

The park is organized around a path stretching between two entry/exit points and connecting various features and destinations.

Gazebo

This is a primary focal point in the park. It provides a sheltered, shaded area with bench seating and accommodates approximately twelve people. The gazebo lends itself to organized as well as informal uses.

Walkways

The concrete sidewalks are wheelchair width to meet accessibility standards; the finish is textured to provide stimulation and to prevent slippage. A wooden bridge was also constructed over a small pond to provide the residents with varying sound and visual stimulation. In selected areas, the pavement widens to form mini-plazas constructed of colored, interlocking bricks.

Artifacts

Several objects, including an old plough, an old-fashioned water pump, and other agricultural implements were integrated into the park to stimulate memories from residents' pasts.

Planters

Several planters are situated throughout the park. The raised planters are made of cedar logs and allow wheelchair access (fig. 2.34). The planters were intended for vegetables and flowers and to provide residents with opportunities to touch, smell, plant and tend, and enjoy the fragrances of various plants.

Figure 2.34
An overview of two accessible planters.

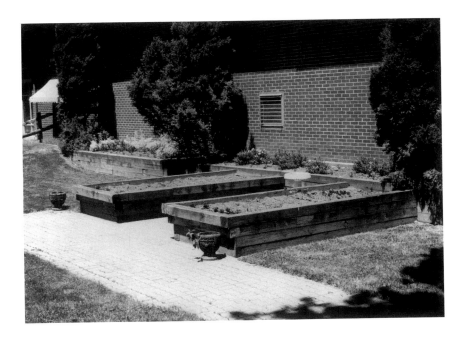

Furnishings

Various types of seating can be found in the garden: benches, swings, and ordinary outdoor chairs (fig. 2.35). Brightly colored awnings were part of the original design, which would have offered shade and enhanced the overall park atmosphere.

Pets

The original plan considered the inclusion of a dog as a year-round resident of the garden. Currently, a bird house is the only provision for animals in the park.

Fencing

Because the building surrounds the park almost entirely, very little fencing is required to complete the secure boundary. This is accomplished with a lattice-type fence and old cedar logs.

Analysis

The overall assessment of the administration is that this park—as well as several other therapeutic parks in regional Niagara—has added to the quality of

Figure 2.35
Various types of seating are placed throughout the park.

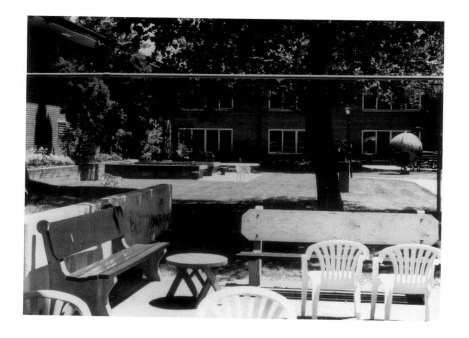

life of residents and encouraged many to become involved in activities and experiences not available indoors.

Several preconditions for success and several shortcomings were identified (Rapelje and Crawford 1987; personal communication, Peter P. Papp, June 1991).

Motivation

There is a need to provide content and social and physical features that will interest and excite residents to go voluntarily to use the outdoors. "People watching" was listed as a primary motivating feature; this finding has direct implications for the design and location of seating arrangements, paths, and activity areas.

Staffing and programmed activities

A certain level of involvement by staff, volunteers, and family members is an additional precondition for success. This involvement can range from highly structured activities conducted by staff to informal participation and "joining" by family members. As in indoor activity spaces, observation of residents for safety is always an added requirement.

The outdoor park provides an opportunity for programming outdoor-specific events such as summer barbecues and other occasions for large, intergenerational gatherings. The atmosphere and quality of these events cannot be replicated in indoor gatherings.

Shortcomings

Several factors hindered full maximization of potential at the outdoor garden in Sunset Haven.

Social Image and Stigma

The label "Therapeutic Park" suggests to both staff and others that this environment was intended as a remedy for a problem, which apparently discourages use by nondemented residents. Through the years, a limited pattern of use has been established, in which the park is used for activities of specific duration, analogous to the indoor activities of "music therapy" or "arts and crafts."

Restricted Physical Access

Sunset Haven's outdoor park was essentially a vacant lot between two buildings, turned into a park. The buildings and their public spaces, such as lounges, dining rooms, and primary circulation paths and doorways, were not designed with the park in mind. The result is a park that has two entry/exit areas at the two furthest points of the facility. While this is an acceptable organization for the park itself, the entry/exit points occur inside the building in fairly inconvenient locations that are hard to identify and locate.

Restricted Visual Access to the Park

For the same reasons outlined above, the park is not visible from most indoor public areas; the visual obscurity further decreases potential use of the park. A major potential for winter use of the park as a visual relief is underutilized.

Therapeutic features   The original features included in Sunset Haven Therapeutic Park were

- countryside agricultural implements
- old gas pump
- sleigh
- gazebo
- pet dog
- bird house
- sundial globe of the world
- raised and stepped planter boxes
- running water course
- old-fashioned lamp posts

The utility and effectiveness of these features vary. First, these features are very different from each other: some have multiple features, such as the gazebo, which is a utilitarian shelter, providing shade and seating; an evocative form; and a defined zone of activity. Other features are primarily a cultural message and a catalyst for reminiscence, such as the gas pump.

The general assessment is that objects and features that are more abstract or out of context, such as the oversized sundial globe, are nonproductive and add visual clutter. "Vernacular" items such as a country water pump and agricultural implements are useful triggers of social interaction and blend well in the landscape. The gazebo and the planters are also successful and have multiple utility. The particular running water course and bridge have been disorienting for residents, and the water course has subsequently been eliminated.

Weiss Institute, Philadelphia Geriatric Center

Address	5301 Old York Road Philadelphia, PA 19141 (215) 456-2000
Owner	Philadelphia Geriatric Center, a member of the Federation of Jewish Agencies
Staff contact	Dr. M. Powell Lawton, Director of Research
Facility type	A research and residential/service special care unit within a major urban geriatric health complex
Residents	Currently a total of 40 residents in stages 2 and 3. There are three 40-bed floors of identical structure.
Staff	Eight nurses, aides, and activity program workers, plus medical personnel and physician assistants
Staff to resident ratio	Approximately 1:4.5
Site/context	A medical campus in an urban context
Date of completion	1972
Size	21,000 square feet (approximate)
Publications	Lawton, M. P., Fulcomer, M., and Kleban, M. H. (1984). Architecture for the mentally impaired elderly. *Environment and Behavior, 16,* pp. 730–737. Leibowitz, B., Lawton, M. P., and Waldman, A. (1979). Evaluation: Designing for impaired elderly people: A prosthetically designed nursing home. *American Institute of Architects Journal, 68,* pp. 59–61.

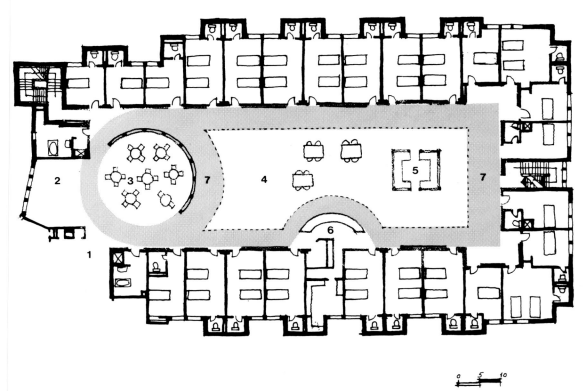

1   secure entry

2   living room

3   dining area

4   activity area

5   gazebo

6   nurses' station

7   wandering path

Sensory Stimulation without Stress

+ One of the primary—and pioneering—premises behind the design of this unit is the assumption that a direct access to stimulation and activities is useful and therapeutic. The open core allows residents to view directly and join any of the activities taking place in the public core.

+ Similarly, the open space allows the staff unobtrusive surveillance of most residents at most times.

— The large open space does not allow acoustical control; at times, unwanted sounds trigger agitation, and the level of noise and disruption leads to further havoc.

Small Activity Clusters

+ The canopied dining area (3), the gazebo for special activities (5), and the common seating area with tables and chairs (2) accommodate a variety of activities and serve to break up the large open space.

Meaningful Wandering Path

+ The wandering path (7) around the perimeter of the public core is another pioneering design feature, allowing continuous movement overlooking activity spaces. The path is integrated with the activity core and eliminates the need for the conventional corridor.

Noninstitutional Environment

— Despite the spatial variety of the public core, its overall character and size are not domestic and familiar.

— The monolithic nurses' station (6) reinforces the institutional image of the unit by its form and the activities that surround it.

— The ceiling grid, lighting fixtures, and lack of daylight and views to the outdoors in the activity core also contribute to the institutional atmosphere.

Background

The Weiss Institute is a 120-bed nursing care unit. The Philadelphia Geriatric Center, the parent institution, is a nonprofit facility consisting of about 520 skilled and intermediate care beds, 500 congregate housing units, a 20-bed accredited geriatric hospital, and a variety of community services for the elderly. About 70 percent of nursing care residents, including those in the Weiss Institute, are on Medicaid.

History: planning a cutting-edge facility

The Weiss Institute opened in 1972 after eight years of planning for both the care and the research programs. The planning process included four national conferences in 1964 and 1966 in which leading gerontologists, service planners, architects, and geriatric physicians provided ideas for the constitution of a care environment for people with Alzheimer's disease. The process continued locally during several years of staff planning, focus groups with residents and relatives, and design of the research to evaluate the eventual plan. Piloting of physical design innovations occurred through the remodeling of several large, multibed rooms into small sleeping areas, buffered from the main hallway by a small social area that afforded both retreat and a simultaneous vantage point for surveying the "action" in the hall.

The results of this exploratory research, coupled with the innovative ideas of psychiatrist consultant Dr. Humphrey Osmond, resulted in the unusual "sociopetal" design of the Weiss Institute. (*Sociopetal* refers to a physical plan that facilitates social interaction.)

Goals
Key therapeutic goals

- Provide a structured therapeutic environment.
- Enhance each resident's sense of self.
- Enhance sensory functioning.
- Increase autonomy in activities of daily living.
- Enhance cognitive functioning and, specifically, memory orientation.
- Increase meaningful use of time.
- Increase social interaction.
- Perform research.

The Weiss Institute originated as the outcome of research on people with dementia in an institutional environment. Findings fed into the planning process through qualitative and quantitative research into the traditional, institutional double-loaded corridor. Left to themselves, residents in these environments crowded into the hallways and congregated near the nurses' station. The conclusion of these studies was that a new design should encourage such congregation but without the crowding and disorder of the eight-foot corridor.

The evaluation of the new design, performed over a several-year period (Lawton, Fulcomer, and Kleban 1984), indicated that some goals were clearly achieved: people used private bedroom spaces and the large, social space to their advantage. The amount of meaningful use of time increased, pathological behavior decreased, and more visiting by relatives was observed. No change in the prevalence of social behavior occurred; because residents had more privacy in the new environment, however, it was concluded that the desired mix of social and private time increased in the aggregate.

Organizational and Social Environment
The staff

Approximately eight staff members operate on the floor at any given time during the day shift. The open plan arrangement allows two or three nurses' aides to supervise most residents visually either from the nurses' station or from critical activity areas.

Program Description

Designated activity periods are scheduled (e.g., music therapy from 3:00 to 4:00 p.m.) and conducted in either secluded area within the large open space. The space itself is an essential aspect of the programming because it is the medium for passive and active behavior, as described below.

Figure 2.37
Overview of the main public space with its various activity zones, surrounded by the wandering path.

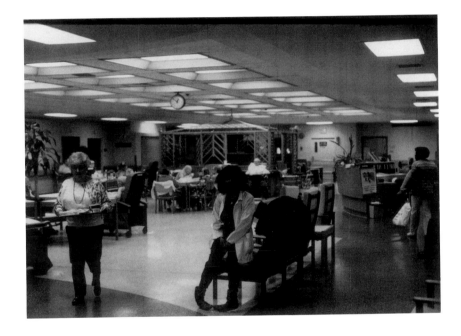

Physical Environment
Description of the plan

The self-contained units occupy the first, second, and third floors of a multistory building. Each unit comprises a large, central, open space, around which residents' rooms are located. The entry zone connects the unit to an elevator and stairs, which lead to other floors and the rest of the building.

The main feature of the design is the large, central area—about forty by sixty feet, including the peripheral pathway—with residents' bedrooms on the outside. This spatial arrangement was adopted for a number of reasons. It serves as a powerful orientational aid for residents, providing visual access to most key areas in the unit from any location. The rationale is that orientation in both time and space is encouraged if the person can see a destination or be reminded of a future event by seeing the place where it will occur. (For example, the sight of the dining area may reinforce time perspective by reminding the person that lunch will be served there.) The earlier research made clear that there was positive value for residents in watching the actions of others, even if purely passively. There is also the chance that positive modeling of normal behavior may occur through watching staff members and others. On a more active level, passive viewers may be motivated to join in activities if they see others participating. Moreover, this arrangement allows staff members unobtrusive surveillance of most residents at most times, usually directly from the nurses' station.

The large open space provides sociopetal areas such as the dining "room," the activity gazebo, areas for structured activities such as music therapy, and informal seating areas in between (fig. 2.37). Availability and easy access to these areas also increases chances of interaction among residents.

The open nature of the plan also provides residents with opportunities to watch other people engaged in various activities. Thus, passive viewers may be encouraged to join in.

Principles of spatial arrangement

The *activity core* is a large, central, rectangular space divided into defined subareas, including a canopied dining area, a common seating area with tables and chairs, and a gazebo for special activities. These elements serve to break up the large space and create spatial variety.

Private/residential spaces surround the central core. There are fifteen double and ten single resident bedrooms. Two bathrooms are located near the entry area.

A *wandering path* around the perimeter of the common space is demarcated by a darker floor covering. This path is free of objects, allowing continuous movement. At the same time, the path is integrated with the activity core and does not constitute a formal corridor.

Surveillance is also a regulating principle of this spatial arrangement and is facilitated by the open plan. Excluding the interior of residents' rooms, visual and auditory surveillance of residents is possible not only from the nurses' station, but also from most points in the unit.

Entry area

All circulation into the unit itself is controlled by a single entry, a "saloon gate" near the elevator lobby, activated by pressing two control buttons simultaneously. Additionally, there are two remote emergency staircases.

Wandering path

The wandering path around the perimeter of the common space is demarcated by a darker floor covering. It serves to separate the private region of residents' rooms from the public activity core. The intention of this design was to facilitate interaction and engage residents in ongoing activities that would be visible from their rooms and from the path when wandering. However, the situation of this public path immediately adjacent to residents' bedrooms may compromise the privacy of these spaces somewhat, as wandering residents travel past residents' private bedrooms. This adjacency also increases the level of noise and distraction in residents' rooms.

Living rooms and social spaces

There is a defined "living room" with a TV set on one side of the central activity space.

Kitchen/dining areas

Dining is facilitated in the unit by the creation of a "dining room" area on one end of the central space (fig. 2.38).

Figure 2.38
A "dining room" defined by a structure within the common public core.

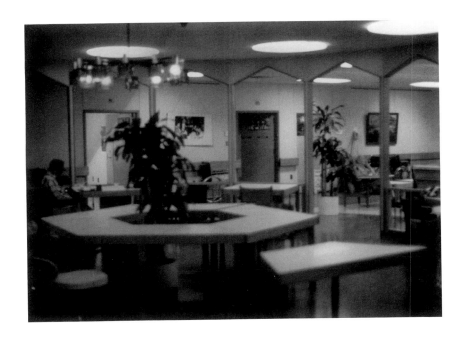

Residents' rooms

There are a total of twenty-five resident rooms, fifteen of which are shared and ten of which are private. Some residents have their own TV in their rooms. The location of residents' rooms adjacent to the wandering path and to the central activity core is intended to draw residents out of their rooms and to engage them to view or participate in activities and social interaction.

Toilet and shower/ tub rooms

Individual rooms include toilets and sinks; bathing facilities are centralized in three large bathrooms, equipped with hydraulic lifts. Two common bathrooms are also located near the entrance.

Materials and surfaces

A vinyl floor is used throughout the unit, with an eight-foot-wide strip of vinyl in a darker tone encircling the periphery of the central open space. Perceptually, this arrangement creates a type of "visual corridor," tying together the doors of the residents' rooms.

The variations in materials, deliberate emphasis on bright colors, liberal use of graphics and textures, and high-level ceiling light combine to provide a relatively high-stimulus-level environment, seen by the sponsors as necessary to counteract the deprivation and underdemand characteristics of the usual institution. This approach contrasts with other approaches to the care of people with Alzheimer's disease, wherein a core aim is reduction of stimulus to reduce anxiety.

The Weiss Institute provides an interesting case study of code expectations. The expectation of a common corridor with physical boundaries is compromised, and the solution retains all of the qualities of the open plan, yet defines a clear and barrier-free path for emergency egress (as well as for wandering).

The unit includes many experimental features, expressed in materials and finishes. Room decor includes color coding through the use of a consistent color scheme for the door seals, bed covers, and other furnishings. Experimental graphics and prominent orienting stimuli act as prostheses for some of the major symptoms of dementia.

Woodside Place

Address	1211 Hulton Road Oakmont, PA 15139
Owner	Presbyterian SeniorCare
Staff contact	Beth Deely, R.N., M.S.N., M.P.M., Director of Alzheimer's Programs, West Penn Hospital and the Presbyterian Association on Aging 1215 Hulton Road Oakmont, PA 15139-1196 (412) 826-6139
Facility type	Freestanding residential Alzheimer's care facility, licensed as a personal care facility; modeled after boarding and personal care homes rather than nursing homes
Residents	Total of 36 residents in three houses of 12 residents each, mostly late stage 1 and stage 2
Staff	Total of 30 full-time-equivalent personnel. This includes a full-time administrator, activity director, and secretary/assistant and a part-time social worker. Other staff include both full- and part-time care attendants, care supervisors, cooks, housekeepers, and maintenance staff. Staff to resident ratio: 1:5 staff to resident ratio from 10:30 a.m. to 7:00 p.m. At other times, the direct staff to resident ratio is 1:9.
Site/context	Located on several acres near a long-term care facility, in a suburban context
Size	23,000 square feet (approximate)
Date of completion	July 1991
Architects	David Hoglund, AIA, Perkins Eastman Architects, New York

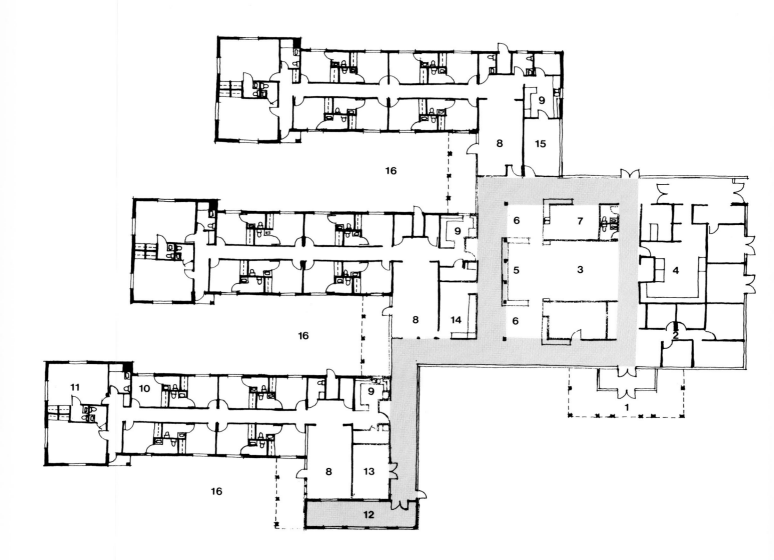

1	entry	
2	administration	
3	great room	
4	main kitchen	
5	fireplace parlor and library	
6	sitting area	
7	country kitchen	
8	living/dining rooms	

9	pantry/serving kitchen
10	single bedroom
11	double bedroom
12	quiet room
13	music room
14	arts and crafts room
15	entertainment room
16	secure courtyards

Variety of Activity Spaces

+ In addition to activity spaces that are integral to each house, a wandering path connects the houses and overlooks a quiet room (*12*), music room (*13*), arts and crafts room (*14*), and entertainment room (*15*). The public core also includes a country kitchen (*7*), sitting areas (*6*), lounge (*5*), and great room (*3*)—certainly sufficient spatial and activity opportunities for the most active and demanding resident.

Figure 2.40
Woodside Place: site map. (Drawing by David Hoglund.)

Positive Outdoor Spaces

+ The design of the outdoor spaces in Woodside is highly integrated with the building: each residential house has its own secure garden, with a sheltered transition space—a terrace—from the living room to the yard. The outer park contains a continuous wandering path and provides larger spaces for both intimate and small group activities, as well as public events (see site map, fig. 2.40).

Meaningful Wandering Path and Circulation

+ The wandering path in this facility is extensive and connects all residential houses with the public core. It overlooks many activity spaces and provides a continuous, donut-shaped path around the great room.
− The path intersects at one corner with the main entry. This has created conflicts severe enough to reconsider the location of the main entry.

− The double rooms at the end of each house are remote destinations, the doors of which are invisible from a distance. These rooms may generate some wayfinding and orientation problems for their residents.

Small Groups of Residents

+ The building block of the facility is the residential house of twelve residents. Each house is a self-contained unit, with its own serving kitchen (*9*), living and dining rooms (*8*), and identifiable entry.

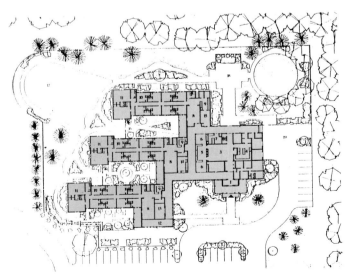

Background
History

In 1988, southwestern Pennsylvania's Allegheny County achieved the dubious distinction of ranking first in the nation in its percentage (22 percent) of adults over the age of sixty. The county also experiences a high concentration of people with Alzheimer's disease.

Also in 1988, the Presbyterian Association on Aging and the Western Pennsylvania Hospital joined together to conduct an investigation of new, more humane ways to care for people with Alzheimer's disease and to fill a gap in the region's care continuum for this population. An eighteen-month study, funded by the Howard Heinz Endowment, allowed a team of geriatric care specialists, health care administrators, and academicians to visit various AD care settings around the United States and in England. The result was Woodside Place—a unique architectural and service concept for providing residential AD care.

Development process

Modeled after "Woodside," a facility in Birmingham, England, Woodside Place houses thirty-six residents with dementia in a residential setting and treats them in a manner significantly different from those housed in nursing or personal care homes. A few of its features are small size; a homelike, personalized setting suitable to wandering safely; the use of "care attendants" specially trained to deal with the unique problems of AD; and Woodside's link to a comprehensive, long-term care continuum. Care approaches include twenty-four-hour, flexible services and secure freedom to wander.

Built to Pennsylvania personal care home standards rather than nursing home standards, Woodside Place eliminates many staffing and building considerations that keep nursing care costs high. The employment of specially trained, nonclinical personnel helps maintain low ongoing operating costs, as does the elimination of many unnecessary structural and equipment items required in nursing home settings.

Funding: financing a demonstration project

Woodside Place is a 2.5-million-dollar project, two million of which was from various foundations and governmental grants. The facility is intended to serve as a demonstration project and is undergoing a three-year, extensive evaluation of its structural design, program, and care components.

Goals
Key therapeutic goals

- *Ensure safety in a nonrestrictive, flexible environment.* For example, secure indoor and outdoor wandering areas have been designed to allow residents to wander independently and safely.
- *Provide a nonstructured schedule and spaces.* Allow residents to function according to "internal" clocks. For example, the common social spaces function in this regard, including the fireplace parlor, the music room, and the kitchen, which is open for around-the-clock use by residents.
- *Maintain homelikeness.* Such administrative decisions as the creation of a comfortable domestic ambience and the use of care attendants rather than nursing home personnel reinforce this goal.

- *Minimize the need for physical and/or chemical restraints.* The freedom of movement and decision making fostered by the design and policies of the facility are intended to reduce resident agitation, therefore decreasing the need for chemical and physical restraints.
- *Maximize residents' coping abilities.* Individually tailored care recognizes residents' strengths and reinforces remaining abilities.
- *Sustain and/or improve clients' orientation, functional abilities, social skills, well-being, and independence.*
- *Provide a stimulating experience for clients* by utilizing visual, auditory, tactile, and olfactory resources to help compensate for sensory loss. One way in which this is done is through careful attention to art work. Interactive art, three-dimensional art, and quilt designs all assist in spatial orientation and reminiscence.
- *Provide for clients along the entire continuum of care.* To this end, a special dementia unit is being developed in the nursing home adjacent to Woodside Place. This sixteen-bed unit will admit residents in the more advanced stages of dementia.

Family goals

- *Increase family caregivers' morale and satisfaction.* This can be accomplished through the relief of some of the caregiver burden through residential and support services. In addition, Woodside provides a monthly family support group and education of caregivers.
- *Provide a cost-effective alternative to nursing home placement.* At approximately 80 percent of nursing home costs, Woodside Place represents a viable, cost effective alternative to nursing home care. In addition, because of the commitment to assist those unable to pay the private rate, 50 percent of Woodside Place residents are low-income individuals.

Program Benefits

The benefits attributed to this milieu include a decreased need for sedatives and tranquilizers, decreased episodes of dysfunctional behaviors (i.e., agitation, anxiety, and combativeness), increased caregiver satisfaction and decreased burden, increased staff morale and decreased turnover, increased resident socialization, and an increased quality of life for residents and families.

Research

The above benefits are being evaluated through a three-year, comprehensive, case-controlled study by principal investigators at the University of Pittsburgh, the Carnegie Mellon University School of Architecture, and the Alzheimer's Disease Research Center. This study will examine and compare residents in three settings—Woodside Place, a traditional nursing home, and a segregated nursing home dementia unit. In addition to this research, a replication manual is under development to be used to assist others developing similar facilities.

Current Status

Woodside Place is the recipient of numerous awards for design; the facility receives frequent inquiries from architects, developers, and professional caregivers throughout North America.

Organizational and Social Environment
The staff

Positions and Ratios

Woodside Place is staffed with an administrator and secretary/assistant, a social worker, licensed practical nurses, an activity director, care attendants, care supervisors, housekeepers, cooks, and maintenance personnel. The budget includes thirty full-time-equivalent personnel. Direct care staff to resident ratios are 1:5 from 10:30 a.m. to 7:00 p.m. and 1:9 at other times.

Organizational Structure and Staffing

The majority of staff members are care attendants who have never worked in a nursing home, substituted for traditional nursing aides. The intention is to staff Woodside with personnel who do not have prior biases about "long-term care" and who will allow residents to live according to their own "internal clocks" and preferences.

Training

The staff of Woodside Place were trained together with volunteers in a three-week, comprehensive training program. This program enhanced team building and included such topics as sleep and AD, sexuality, first aid, body system changes with aging, problem solving for difficult behaviors, and delivering activity programs. Training included national and local speakers, films, family and nurse panels, and experiential learning through site visits to adult day care centers and one-on-one experience with people with dementia.

Ongoing staff development and education are also provided on a monthly basis, and a staff learning manual has been developed to train new employees as the need arises.

The residents

Characteristics of the Residents

Woodside Place filled to capacity within a month and a half of opening. Currently, twenty-four women and twelve men reside in the facility. The average age is eighty-one, and residents are sixty-three to ninety-three years old.

Admission and Retention

Admission and discharge criteria for Woodside Place were carefully developed and shared with family caregivers prior to entry. To be admitted, residents were required to have a geriatric assessment. This was required for all initial residents, but, because of the varying quality of assessments, it is currently encouraged only. In its place, the social worker conducts in-home assessments and reports her findings to an admission team composed of the geriatrician, social worker, administrator, and geriatric clinical nurse specialist. Because of the facility's strong link with West Penn Hospital, medical care and expertise are readily available.

Physical Environment
Description of the plan

Each house is self-contained with its own sleeping, dining, and social areas for family-like interactions—subscribing to familiar, home-like settings. The houses and shared areas (music room, fireplace parlor, library, and activities kitchen) are connected by meandering corridors that allow residents to wander freely. The structure is surrounded by additional, secured, outdoor wandering paths, accessed through the patio gardens of each house. The sloped roof pattern emphasizes individual houses.

Principles of spatial arrangement

- The plan is divided into *three houses.*
- Central *social spaces and an internal wandering street* connect all three houses.
- Within each household, *residents' rooms are organized around the outdoor courtyard and natural area* to provide visual access to the outdoors from every room.

Entry area

A circular drive is designed for caregivers to drop residents off at the sheltered doorway. Upon entering the facility, one steps into a large vestibule, situated between the wandering path and the secretary/reception area. Straight ahead, the great room attracts residents, and the internal wandering street leads residents to both individual households and common social spaces.

Outdoor spaces

Individual garden courtyards are associated with and accessible from each of the households. These south-facing courtyards serve as places to wander freely, garden, eat outdoors, and enjoy nature. All three courtyards open to a larger, common outdoor area, also designed for wandering independently and experiencing the outdoors. An additional shared courtyard contains raised planters for gardening, and an adjacent covered veranda functions as an outdoor room for wandering and outdoor activities in light rain or hot sun. All residents' rooms have visual access to one or more of these outdoor spaces.

Staff "retreat" or lounge areas

Administrative spaces are grouped together at the northern end of the facility. These include a secretary/reception room, four offices (including one for the research team), supply storage and support services, a staff lounge, and a conference room.

Wandering paths

An indoor, meandering, secure wandering path linking households and common social spaces—conceived as an internal street—has been provided for use by residents at all times. Outdoor wandering paths in the courtyards and larger grounds were also designed for independent resident use.

Residents' rooms

Two double rooms and eight single rooms are provided in each household. Each room has a direct view to an outdoor courtyard or natural area. Each resident has his or her own closet, and each resident's room has a sink and toilet.

Toilet and shower/ tub rooms

Toilet rooms are located in each resident room. One or two showers are situated in each household as well. A room for a whirlpool bath is also located in the common area.

Kitchen/dining areas

In addition to the central activity kitchen where meals are cooked for all of the households, a country kitchen for resident use on a twenty-four-hour basis is situated in the central common area, adjacent to the internal wandering street. This kitchen is used by residents, families, and volunteers for making beverages and snacks and socializing over a cozy kitchen table.

Each house also has its own small area for dining, with four square tables for three people each. Because residents eat according to their own schedules, this space is usually occupied by at least a few residents snacking or enjoying a meal at all times.

Social and quiet spaces

The *great room* is the one great gathering space for all residents. It is a place for wandering, holiday meals and special celebrations, visiting, exercise classes, live performances, movies, and games. This room is intended to be noisy and filled with people at some times and quiet with small-group activities at others.

The *fireplace parlor and library*—intended to emulate the heart and hearth of home life—is a place for informal conversation, quiet reading and games, and visiting with family members and friends. It is intended to serve as a visual reference point from all of the public areas of the facility and will house current and historical periodicals, newspapers, and books for residents' enjoyment.

The *oasis room* is a quiet space at the end of the internal wandering path. It is a place for quiet solitude, to pace, slow down, and avoid distractions.

Each individual household also has its own living/dining room area, with informal seating and dining tables for household activities.

Activity spaces

The *music room* is a parlorlike room along the internal wandering street. It houses a player piano and other instruments and equipment for making music and sound.

Residents' laundry rooms are located adjacent to the country kitchen and in each house.

The *crafts lounge* is a niche full of fabrics, paper goods, textures, and textile patterns. It is a place to sew, knit, and share one's hobby; to browse through drawers and cupboards; and to display crafts and seasonal articles.

An *entertainment room* houses a large-screen TV and VCR for watching old movies or sports events in a cozy, living room–like environment.

Alexian Village of Milwaukee

Address	Alexian Village Health Center 9255 North 76th Street Milwaukee, WI 53223 (414) 355-9300
Owner	Alexian Brothers Healthcare System
Staff contact	Daniel C. Krejci, President
Facility type	Continuum of care retirement community with a 61-bed skilled nursing facility and respite center for both people with dementia and others
Residents	A total of 398 residents currently reside in the independent living apartments. The Health Center provides 61 beds for both short-term recuperation/ rehabilitation and long-term residential use. A new 87-bed Health Center is currently under construction; this building will include two floors of resident rooms. A day care unit will also be included in the new facility, as will spaces for some health care services. In the current Health Center, 18 percent of the residents are admitted for short-term recuperation/rehabilitation. The remainder are long-term residents, of whom 83 percent are memory impaired, and most demonstrate low levels of functional ability. Residents are assigned to units on the basis of behavioral characteristics and medical condition.
Staff	Registered nurse manager for each floor, registered and licensed practical nurses, nursing assistants, activity and social service personnel
Staff to resident ratio	1:6 during the day shift (7:00 a.m. to 3:00 p.m.); 1:7 on the evening shift (3:00 p.m. to 11:00 p.m.); 1:11 on the night shift (11:00 p.m. to 7:00 a.m.)
Site/context	23-acre suburban campus in the northwestern corner of Milwaukee
Size (approximate)	Alexian Village campus: 23 acres Health Center: 70,000 square feet, total building; 19,100 square feet on each residential floor
Date of completion	Alexian Village was established in 1980; the construction of a new Health Center building is scheduled for completion in August 1992.
Architects	Ellerbe Becket, St. Paul, Minnesota Holland & Steed, Deerfield, Illinois Lorainne Hiatt, Design Consultant

Figure 2.41   Plan of the Alexian Village of Milwaukee, Wisconsin.

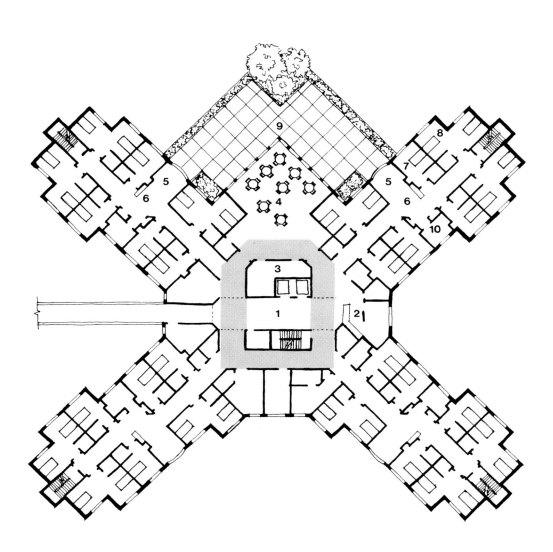

1	entry area	**6**	work station
2	central nursing station	**7**	single room
3	serving kitchen	**8**	double room
4	dining room	**9**	secure outdoor patio
5	living rooms	**10**	cluster shower room

CONTEMPORARY ENVIRONMENTS FOR PEOPLE WITH DEMENTIA

Small Groups of Residents

\+ Ten residents are grouped in seven rooms to create an identifiable cluster. Each household has its own living room, with a noninstitutional service nurses' desk.

Positive Outdoor Space

\+ The patio is a generous outdoor extension of the dining room and a visual relief for two lounges. Its size provides the potential for creative and meaningful use of the space even on above-ground floors.

Circulation Spaces

− The central core—stairs, elevators, and associated circulation—is large and unobstructed and may be perceived as institutional. Most circulation paths are not associated with any activities and are potentially disorienting.

Residents' Rooms

The plan provides a mix of three double rooms and four single rooms for each household.

\+ The double room configuration—an L shape—is an elegant solution for spatial separation and the provision of some privacy and a sense of ownership. Each resident's room has a toilet and a sink.

Activity Spaces

\+ There are a variety of activity spaces in the facility: lounges, activity room, patio, assembly room, chapel, and beauty parlor.

− The floor illustrated has a very large dining room for forty residents in an undifferentiated space.

Cedar Acres Adult Day Center

Address	1930 South River Road Janesville, WI 53546
Owner	Cedar Crest
Staff contact	Myra Kobs, M.S.W., Director
Facility type	Day care
Participants	Maximum of 24; daily average of approximately 21
Staff	Full-time nurse, cook, director/social worker, clerical staff members, aides, and activity director; part-time financial advisor
Staff to resident ratio	1:4
Site/context	Renovated 100-year-old farmhouse on a seven-acre site in rural southwestern Wisconsin
Size (approximate)	3,520 square feet on the ground floor 800 additional square feet of second floor office space
Date of completion	House built in the 1800s; the addition of an activity room was completed in 1989.
Architects	Addition designed by Jim Cullen Inc., Wisconsin. Original architect of home unknown. Production drawings by Potter Design Group, Madison, Wisconsin

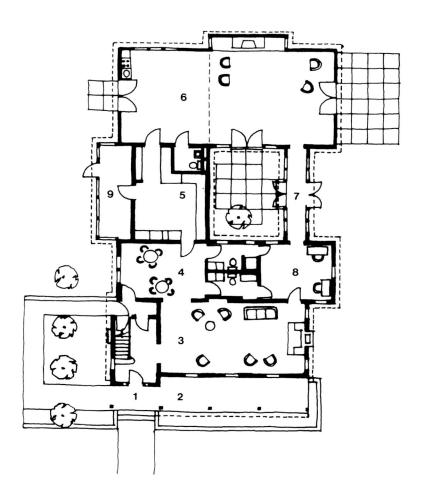

1   entrance

2   porch

3   living room

4   dining room

5   kitchen

6   partitioned activity room (an addition)

7   breezeway

8   office

9   screened porch

Noninstitutional Image

\+ Despite the large number of users and caregivers at peak time —close to twenty-five— the place has a perfect domestic and residential atmosphere.

Variety of Activity Spaces

\+ The house has numerous activity spaces of various sizes and moods, and it can accommodate several simultaneous activities.

Positive Outdoor Spaces

\+ The house has a secure, large outdoor garden, bird feeders, bushes planted in memory of people, and seating.

\+ An adjacent structure accommodates a horse boarded at the center, a catalyst for numerous activities.

\+ The open, landscaped front yard is also used by residents who are not wanderers.

Tapping Local Resources

\+ Because of its location, staff members take advantage of various "rural" events and conduct frequent outings.

Circulation

\− The circulation through the house requires passage through activity spaces to reach other spaces. The circulation is disorienting, and central monitoring of residents is often difficult.

Stimulation

\− Because of the interconnectedness of most spaces, it is difficult to control the level of stimulation or prevent disruptions.

Figure 2.43
Cedar Acres Adult Day Center, exterior view.

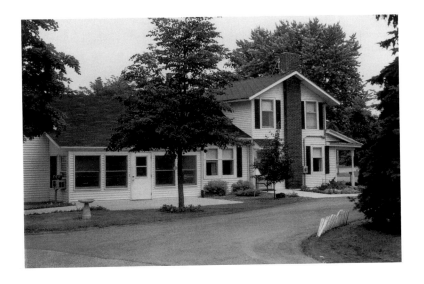

Elderkare

Address	2086 Colony Court Beloit, WI (608) 221-1944
Owner	Community Care Alternatives
Staff contact	Delores M. Moyer, President, Community Care Alternatives
Facility type	Community-based group home for 12 residents
Residents	A total of 12 residents, 11 of whom are women. Most residents or their children are from the local area. Residents come to the home from nursing homes, family members' homes, and other group homes. (This is the first dementia-specific group home in the area.)
Staff	Geriatric nurse practioner, resident aides, and a weekly beautician
Staff to resident ratio	1:4, with each staff member directly responsible for four specific residents
Site/context	Suburban, multifamily housing residential area
Size	5,200 square feet (approximate)
Date of completion	February 1991
Architects	Design by Delores Moyer and George Noll Linville Design
Publication	New facilities planned for Alzheimer's patients. (1990). *Mature Lifestyles,* September.

Figure 2.44   Plan of Elderkare, Beloit, Wisconsin.

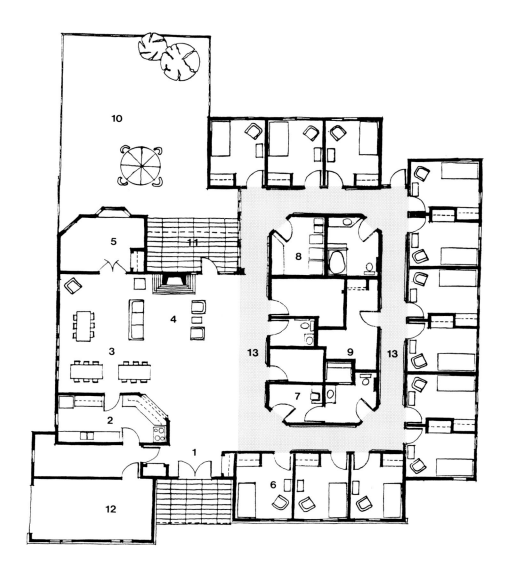

1 entry	**8** laundry
2 kitchen	**9** office and storage area
3 dining area	**10** secure garden
4 living area	**11** sheltered patio
5 den	**12** garage
6 resident's room	**13** wandering path
7 beauty parlor	

Noninstitutional Image

\+ In addition to its single story, pitched roof, fireplace chimney, and single-car garage, the residential image of the facility is enhanced by the domestic image of the interior spaces.

Wandering Path

\+ Despite the fact that the path around the service core is largely a conventional corridor, the institutional image of the path is diminished in part by the cut corners and the open views at both ends into the public area.

— The emergency door at the end of the corridor is a tempting target for wandering residents.

Variety of Activity Areas

\+ The relatively small building includes many resident activity spaces: living room, dining space, den, laundry room, beauty parlor, kitchen, patio, and outdoor garden.

— The kitchen provides limited visual access to public spaces.

Interior Finishes

\+ Each hallway is color coded, the furnishings are moisture-proof (and yet noninstitutional), and each room has a unique set of curtains, wallpaper, and paintings.

Positive Outdoor Space

The outdoor space is still an underdeveloped, grass yard.

\+ The covered patio provides a degree of shelter and a positive microclimate.

Director's Office

— The original location of the office was a small room facing the activity space, which provided insufficient privacy. The current location is a room that is also used for linen storage and is perhaps too private.

Other Observations

All rooms are single occupancy.
By policy, there are no private toilet rooms.
Public bath rooms are wheelchair accessible.

Hale Kako'O (House to Uphold and Support)

Address	Alewa Heights Respite Center 2200 Block, Alewa Drive Honolulu, HI
Owner	City and County of Honolulu and the Alzheimer's Association, Honolulu Chapter
Staff contact	Laurie Meininger, Executive Director Alzheimer Association, Honolulu Chapter (808) 521-3771
Facility type	Day and short-term respite care center
Residents	12 day care clients and 12 additional overnight respite residents
Staff	Six staff members (day), two staff members (night)
Staff to resident ratio	1:4 (day); 1:6 (night)
Site/context	Urban residential neighborhood; single family housing area on a hill, with a panoramic view of Honolulu
Size (approximate)	2,700 square feet Additional 1,800 square feet for lower level office, meeting, and storage space
Date of completion	Under development; expected completion in 1992
Architects	Design Partners Inc., Honolulu; Owen Chock, Principal
Design consultants	Uriel Cohen and Gerald Weisman, Milwaukee, Wisconsin

Figure 2.45   Plan of Hale Kako'O, Honolulu, Hawaii.

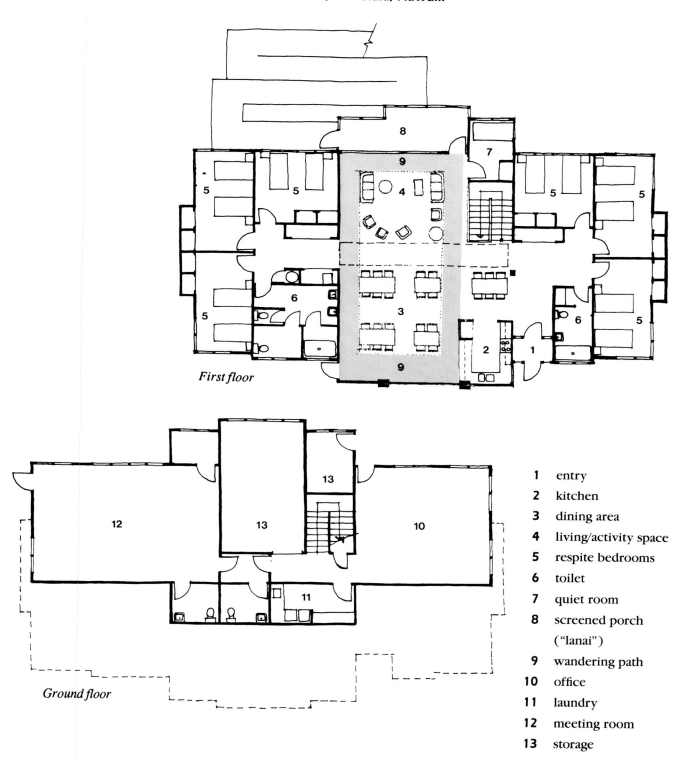

First floor

Ground floor

1 entry
2 kitchen
3 dining area
4 living/activity space
5 respite bedrooms
6 toilet
7 quiet room
8 screened porch
   ("lanai")
9 wandering path
10 office
11 laundry
12 meeting room
13 storage

Noninstitutional Image

+   The size of the house and its form are typical of houses in this neighborhood.

Staying Dry

—   Although they are provided in accordance with state day care regulations, the number and location of the toilet rooms may not be adequate for peak day use. While toilet rooms on the lower level can also be used if necessary, these are inconvenient and the change in levels is probably impossible for participants to negotiate cognitively.

Usable Circulation and Discrete Entry

+   The simple plan provides direct visual access to most destinations, yet discreetly buffers the entry from the interior public space.

Unobtrusive Surveillance

+   The open plan and compact public space allow unobtrusive monitoring from the kitchen or other activity points to almost all public parts of the building.

Size

—   Although domestic and residential in scale, the public space is too small for the peak attendance of twenty-four persons.

Domestic Ambience

+   The internal organization of the plan is basically domestic, with a familiar kitchen-dining-living room connection.

—   The lack of subspaces and the crowded formation of the dining room furniture may contribute to an institutional ambience.

Wandering Path

+   Despite the compact organization of the plan, it provides a coherent wandering path that is an integral part of the dining and living room.

+   This plan is essentially without corridors.

Helen Bader Center, Milwaukee Jewish Home

Address	1414 North Prospect Milwaukee, WI 53202 (414) 276-2627
Owner	Milwaukee Jewish Home
Staff contact	Nita Corré, Executive Director
Facility type	Community-based group home attached to several residential and service facilities for the elderly
Residents	24 residents, Stage 2, high to moderate level of functioning
Staff	Two full-time staff members and various part-time personnel for specific programs and administration
Staff to resident ratio	1:12 direct care (full-time paid employees); actually 1:6 including full time volunteer employees
Site/context	The Bader Center completes the continuum of care campus provided by the Milwaukee Jewish Home. The urban setting includes a mid-rise, independent and assisted living building with community services, all connected to an existing skilled care facility.
Size	16,000 square feet (approximate)
Date of completion	Presently an advanced schematic design. Completion and occupancy are anticipated in late 1993.
Architects	Kahler Slater, Architects, Milwaukee, Wisconsin
Design consultants	Uriel Cohen and Gerald Weisman; Nita Corré

Figure 2.46   Plan of the Helen Bader Center, Milwaukee, Wisconsin.

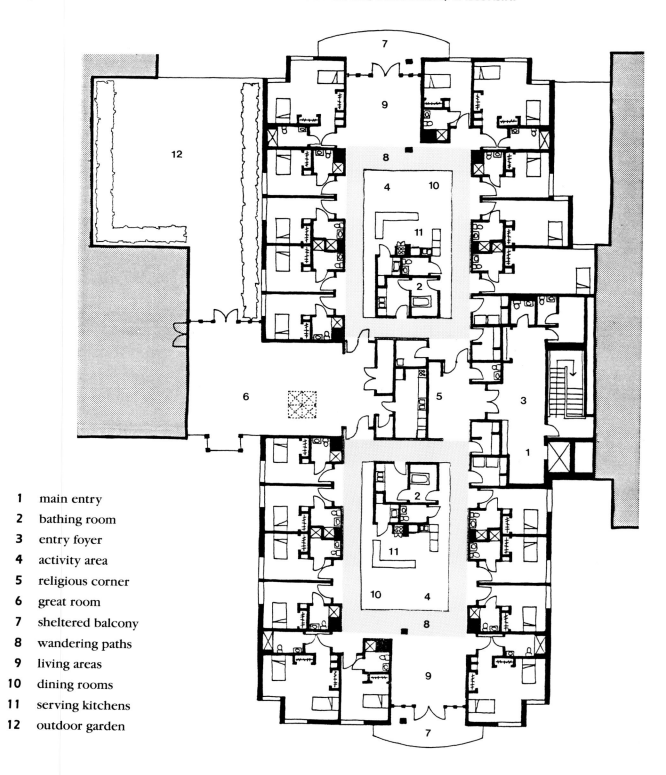

1 main entry
2 bathing room
3 entry foyer
4 activity area
5 religious corner
6 great room
7 sheltered balcony
8 wandering paths
9 living areas
10 dining rooms
11 serving kitchens
12 outdoor garden

Things from the Past

+   A special activity space (5) has a religious corner with objects and decor with long-time meaning to most current residents. This space can serve as a catalyst for reminiscence as well as a functional space for small-group religious practice.

Variety of Activity Spaces

+   In addition to activity spaces in the residential cluster, simultaneous activities can take place in other shared spaces: (3) the entry foyer; (6) great room; sheltered balconies (7); and (12) the outdoor garden.

Smaller Groups of Residents

+   The unit is divided into two small households of twelve residents each; both clusters have their own living, dining, and activity spaces.

Design for Changing Needs

+   The floor plan allows a variety of space uses: the two households can be connected or separated, and the great room (6) can be accessible to either or both households.

Tapping Local Resources

+   The decision to locate this group home on a crowded urban campus was largely influenced by the desire to relate to local resources, places, and people. The adjacent buildings offer a variety of activity spaces and events (e.g., a synagogue and a kosher delicatessen restaurant).

Noninstitutional Image

The unit is attached to a complex of large midrise buildings.
+   A major effort was made to keep the scale of the unit small, to give it a clear and separate identity when viewed from the street, and to decrease the institutional image of the unit.

Entry and Transition

−   Because of its location on the second floor and the connection of the entry to an existing building with its own underground parking, the whole entry and transition experience is indirect, lengthy, and potentially disorienting to visitors and residents alike.

John Douglas French Center for Alzheimer's Disease

Address	3951 Katella Avenue Los Alamitos, CA 90720
Owner	National Medical Enterprises, Inc.
Staff contact	Ferri Kidane, Executive Director
Facility type	Three-story, freestanding facility specifically designed to accommodate people with dementias and similar disorders. This facility provides longitudinal, integrated services for all stages of the disease. Services include long-term care, short-term respite care, social day care, outpatient diagnostic assessment and geriatric case management, and clinical research.
Residents	148 long-term care residents reside in six care units, assigned according to nursing care needs, cognitive abilities, and behavioral tendencies. Twenty-five participants attend the day care program.
Staff	Full-time geropsychiatrist medical director, licensed family counselor, social worker, therapeutic recreational therapist and a team of certified activities' directors, registered dietician, nursing team comprising a director of nursing services, an assistant director, and an R.N. on each shift, L.P.N.s and certified nursing assistants, outpatient clinic director (R.N.), and adult day care director.
Staff to resident ratio	1:5 days; 1:7 evenings; 1:12 nights
Site/context	Located along a major artery in Los Alamitos, a southern California suburb 30 miles south of Los Angeles
Size	74,000 square feet (approximate)
Date of completion	Fall 1987
Architects	Stevens & Wilkinson, Inc., Atlanta, Georgia
Publications	French, D. K., and Eamer, R. K. (1987). Center for Alzheimer's patients one-of-a-kind. *American Health Care Association's Provider for Long Term Care Professionals,* November. Stevens, P. S. (1987). Design for dementia: Recreating the loving family. *American Journal of Alzheimer's Care and Research,* January/February, 16–22. Bowe, J. (1988). State-of-the-art Alzheimer's facilities take the lead in scientific research. *Today's Nursing Home and Retirement Housing Today Quarterly, 9* (8), 1, 6–7.

Figure 2.47

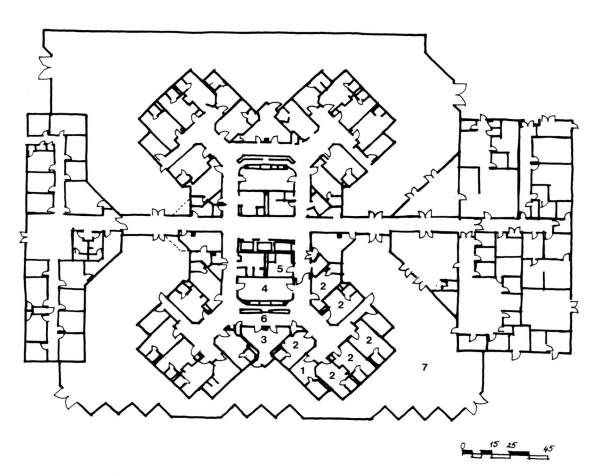

1   resident's room—one bed

2   resident's room—two beds

3   activities area

4   dining area

5   bathroom

6   nurses' station

7   courtyard

Variety of Activity Areas

— Because of California regulatory code restrictions and other constraints, many of the butterfly concept features were not maximized in this facility: the integral activity/dining area was reduced to an activity area (3) shared by two clusters, and the dining area was moved to a large, interior room.

Noninstitutional Image

— The reduction in social amenities contributed to an institutional image, reinforced by substantial nurses' stations in prominent locations and by the overall monolithic scale of the three-story building, which is evident despite the division into small units.

Wandering Path

— The size of the facility and code restrictions generated a plan with a substantial interior core, which is surrounded by a conventional, double-loaded corridor that intersects other paths. Although continuous wandering is possible, the potential for confusion, disorientation, and conflict with activities is high.

Small Groups of Residents

+ The most visible aspect of the butterfly concept in this facility is the creation of small clusters of thirteen residents in each. The residential cluster is the building block of the facility.

The generic butterfly plan, designed by Stevens and Wilkinson, was an important development.

+ It promoted the concept of small groups of residents. This configuration creates identifiable clusters, each with its own social and activity spaces (*2*). The institutional corridor is diminished, and a secure courtyard or patio (*4*) provides secure outdoor space for varied activities.

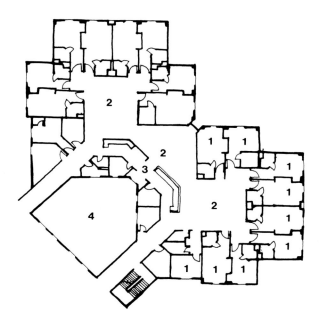

1 residents' rooms
2 activity/dining areas
3 nurses' station
4 courtyard or patio

Namesté Alzheimer Center

Address	2 Penrose Boulevard Colorado Springs, CO 80906 (719) 475-2000
Owner	Penrose-St. Francis Health Care Systems
Staff contact	Moira Reinhardt, Administrator
Facility type	Freestanding long term care facility, with an adjoining day care facility on the ground floor
Residents	Total of 60 residents in four "pods" of 15 residents each; 30 residents require only custodial care, 15 require intermediate care, and 15 require skilled nursing care.
Staff	R.N. administrator, director of nursing, activity therapist, coordinator of volunteers, social worker, two activity aides, R.N.s, and certified nursing assistants (based on activities), part-time dietician, and daily volunteers
Staff to resident ratio	Approximately 1:5 during the day (7:00 a.m. to 11:00 p.m.); 1:11 at night (11:00 p.m. to 7:00 a.m.)
Site/context	A building on a large, suburban, residential site on the outskirts of Colorado Springs, overlooking the mountains
Charges	$88 per day for semiprivate rooms and $103 per day for private rooms
Size	40,000 square feet (approximate)
Date of completion	1990
Architects	Randy Thorn, Architects, Colorado Springs, Colorado

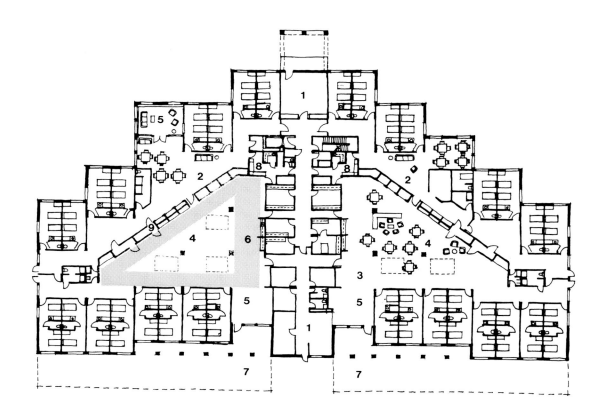

1 entrances
2 units for more dependent residents
3 units for more active residents
4 public core: dining area, living area, serving kitchen, and activity spaces
5 den/sun room
6 wandering path
7 secure outdoor space
8 nurses' station
9 storage wall

Aging in Place

+ The four residential clusters allow grouping of residents with four different levels of abilities and provide for internal shifts of residents due to changing needs.

Activity Alcoves

+ The two large residential clusters offer more complex and varied public space and a greater range of public to private spaces: the central dining and living areas are open and exposed; the den (5) is more private and overlooks an outdoor extension.

− The activity core in each larger unit is basically windowless, despite the skylights. Large, undifferentiated open space is typically considered nonresidential.

Wandering Path

+ The two larger units provide a continuous wandering path, which overlooks activity spaces. These two units are essentially corridorless. All pods have doors that open to the paths.

Unobtrusive, Centralized Surveillance

+ One nursing station/office (8) serves as a visual control point for two adjacent units, unobtrusively monitoring thirty-two residents in these units.

Residents' Rooms

− The two occupants of each room in the larger units are separated by centrally located toilet rooms; the "outer" occupant has a private space, while the "inner" occupant is enclosed in a less private space with no view to the exterior.

Figure 2.50
Namesté Alzheimer Center, exterior view.

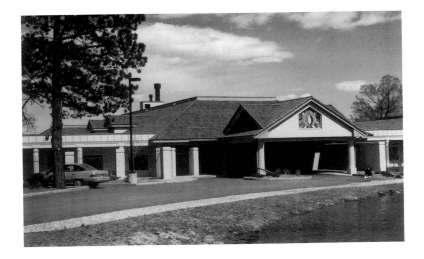

Stonefield Home

Address	6701 Stonefield Road Middleton, WI 53562 (608) 831-2707
Owner	Alternative Living Services
Staff contact	Laura Bartell, Community Services Representative
Facility type	Specially designed, community-based residential facility serving elderly residents in various stages of dementia. Stonefield Home is one of eleven facilities operated in Wisconsin by Alternative Living Services.
Residents	There are twenty-four residents, most of whom are experiencing confusion and incontinence and require assistance with most activities of daily living. A majority of residents come from other assisted living facilities, retirement homes, or nursing homes.
Staff	R.N. director, community services representative, full-time recreational therapist, full- and part-time cooks, plus a care-giving staff on all three shifts. There is also an interdisciplinary team of professionals that service all Alternative Living Services facilities. A visiting beautician and podiatrist come to the home on a weekly basis.
Staff to resident ratio	1:6 (first and second shift); 1:12 (third shift)
Site/context	Newly developed suburban residential area
Size	14,000 square feet (approximate)
Date of completion	March 1991
Architects	Eugene Guskowski, Shepard Legan Aldrian Architects

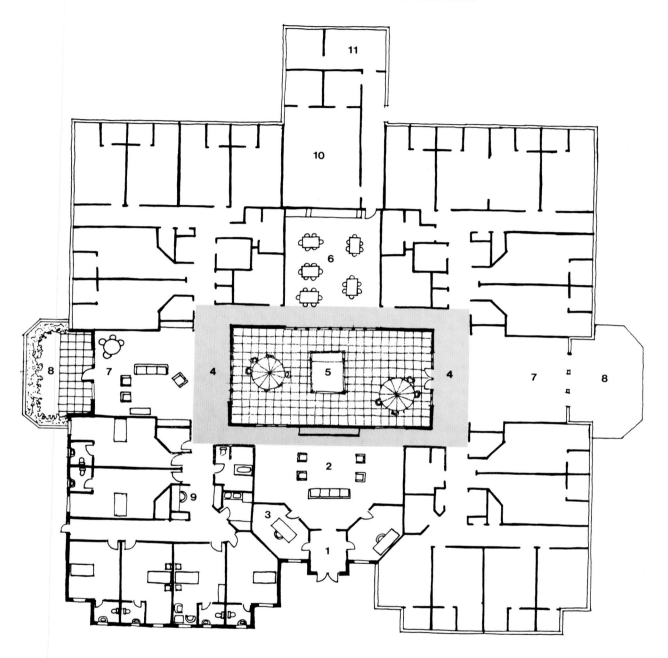

1	entry foyer	5	open courtyard	9	nurses' station
2	living room	6	dining room	10	kitchen
3	office	7	living rooms	11	staff
4	wandering path	8	secure gardens/patios		

Noninstitutional Image

+ The organization of the public spaces around the interior court and the integration of the wandering path (4) with these spaces eliminate the conventional institutional corridor from this zone.

+ The nurses' stations (9) in each residential cluster are very modest, domestic, and informal work stations in a wall nook.

– The common dining room is very large; despite the domestic decor, it is not intimate. The kitchen is totally separate from the residents' "home range"—a waste of a potentially important activity space.

Meaningful Wandering Path

+ The wandering path (4) that surrounds the interior courtyard is an integral part of the public space; the continuous path overlooks many activities and provides visual interest and stimulation in both the summer and the winter.

Small Groups of Residents

+ The unit is divided into four residential clusters.

– Two clusters share one living/activity room (7). The spatial organization of the living room does not maximize its potential as an integral front of the cluster, contributing to its identity.

Positive Outdoor Space

+ The central outdoor courtyard (5) is a major organizing element of the floor plan; it provides daylight to all primary interior spaces and aids in orientation.

+ The courtyard is secure and can accommodate both formal and informal activities.

+ The side yards/patios (8) are additional activity spaces associated with the living rooms. They provide degrees of shelter and offer a positive microclimate.

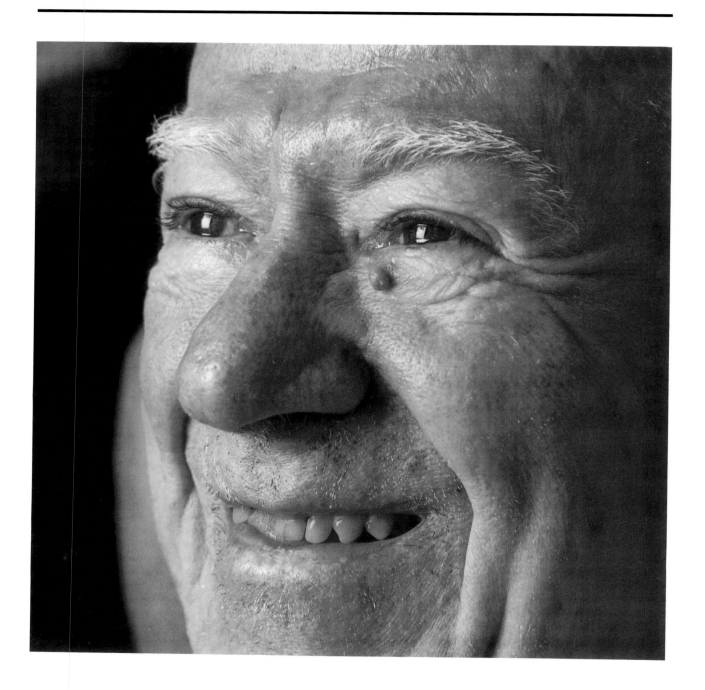

3   Critical Issues and Concepts

This integrative chapter addresses selected key issues and problems of people with dementia and their formal and informal caregivers. Lessons and examples from various case studies are used to illustrate and substantiate design concepts or approaches to physical and programmatic solutions.

A number of topics remain controversial; different respondents report widely disparate views and experiences. Many of these topics represent subjects for systematic research. Others are simply issues for decision making founded on a value-based world view and an informed philosophy of care.

Aging in Place

According to the Dictionary of Gerontology (Harris 1988), *aging in place* refers to "the effect of time on a nonmobile population; remaining in the same residence where one has spent his or her earlier years" (p. 18). More specifically, aging in place normally refers to the ideal condition of not having to leave one's home environment as a consequence of insufficient support services to respond to changing needs. Such changes are most frequently deteriorating health, death of spouse, or loss of income (Pastalan 1990). The onset or progression of dementia is such a change in health—one that frequently precedes a move from one's own home in the community to an institution, or that requires an increase in the level or type of care needed, with a consequent change in living arrangements. Aging in place is commonly promoted as a strategy for maintaining autonomy, independence, sense of identity, and quality of life, as well for maximizing financial resources.

In addition to the idea of remaining within one's familiar home and community, *aging in place* may also refer to residential life away from home: it is the concept of remaining within the same facility or facilities throughout various stages of dementia, alleviating the need for frequent moves and difficult reorientation as the disease progresses. This second type of aging in place can be further subdivided into (1) aging in place despite changes in needs for services and consequent living arrangements and level of care (e.g., remaining on the same campus, which provides a continuum of care as needs progress from day care to group home to long-term care) and (2) aging in place within a setting that provides a particular level of care (e.g., remaining in the same long-term care setting) throughout various stages of the disease, without the need to relocate to more "advanced" facilities as conditions deteriorate.

Little is actually known about the possible benefits and detriments of aging in place (in the sense of remaining in one's own home) for people with dementia, although the idea is instinctively attractive and is endorsed by many authors (Cohen and Weisman 1991). The concept of aging in place in one's own home may have specific consequences when applied to people with dementia, as their condition and level of access to services also affects the ability of their caregiver(s) to continue to enjoy life in the home and community. Aging in place in the home—particularly in the context of people with dementia—should not be pursued fanatically, as the choice of *if* and *when* a person with dementia should relocate is a highly subjective—personal—and family decision. The issue of aging in place in the home among people with dementia warrants conclusive future research.

The two additional conceptions of aging in place—(1) aging in place, the continuity between levels of care and living arrangements, and (2) aging in place within a single living arrangement that accommodates various levels of care—are further discussed and analyzed below to highlight particular advantages and disadvantages and to explore possible environmental implications of these ideas.

Many of the facilities examined offered more than a single service or level of care. For example, several group homes and long term care facilities also accommodate day and/or respite care. This arrangement can provide many benefits for the person with dementia, the caregiver(s), and the facility staff and administration, including continuity of care, a familiar environment and staff, reduced time needed for orientation and familiarization, and greater awareness of the residents' individual habits, preferences, and needs.

One example of such a facility is the Alzheimer Care Center in Gardiner, Maine. In addition to the twenty-eight residents served by the boarding home, the facility accommodates an additional six to eight day care clients and up to two respite care residents at a time. The relationship between day, respite, and boarding home care has had positive implications for residents, family members, and staff. Most of the boarding home residents were introduced to the facility via the day care and respite programs, a fact that has greatly reduced the amount of time necessary for adjustment to the facility for residents and family members. In fact, residents who enter the facility after having participated in one or both of these programs take less time and have fewer negative experiences during orientation to the facility than do residents who had not previously participated in day care or respite here, according to staff members. Administrators now recommend that all potential boarding home residents participate in either the day care or respite program.

This participation acts additionally as a trial period for both the resident and family and the staff. Families can evaluate the facility, the staff, and their family member during and subsequent to participation in day care or respite and decide whether the center is the most appropriate setting for their family member. Staff members are also given the opportunity for a thorough assessment of the resident before admission, to ascertain whether he or she is appropriately suited to the center.

Finally, the relationship between day/respite care and the boarding home has positive financial implications for the center, as participants in these services represent a natural pool of potential residents for the boarding home.

Another example is the Alois Alzheimer Center, which provides dementia specific day care and short-term respite in addition to a residential program that accommodates eighty-two residents. In addition, for those in the residential program, the facility is divided into three sections, which physically and programmatically respond to the needs of the individuals who reside in each section. As a person changes, progresses, or improves in the disease, he or she is moved into other areas of the facility, which are altered (environment, programs, and staffing) and thus better suited to meet individual needs. This arrangement promotes the highest level of functioning for each individual without denying those with greater capabilities a more stimulating environment because other residents are unable to cope.

The Pathways Project of the Miami Jewish Home and Hospital for the Aged, in Miami, Florida, is a facility designed for aging in place and continuity over changes in necessary level of care (fig. 3.1). This continuum of care campus—

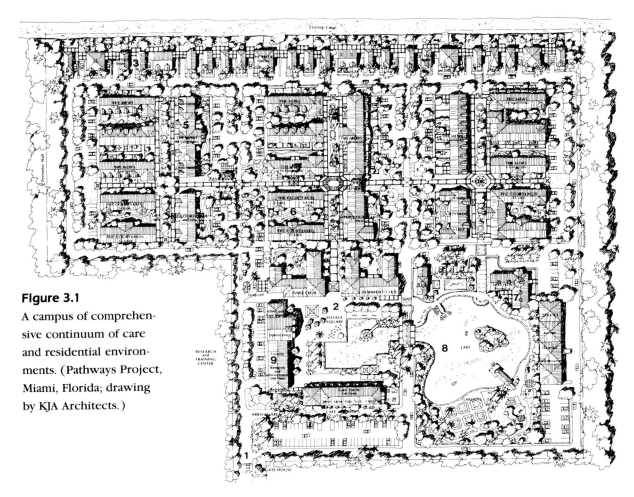

Figure 3.1
A campus of comprehensive continuum of care and residential environments. (Pathways Project, Miami, Florida; drawing by KJA Architects.)

currently in the planning stage—will offer day and respite care, home care, assisted living apartments, congregate housing apartments, group homes, long-term care, a hospice, and cooperative houses for caregivers. Each living arrangement responds to a required level of care, as well as to individual preferences for privacy and independence. Ideally, people with dementia and their caregivers will continue to live comfortably on the campus through both the intermediate and the late stages of the disease, and caregivers will continue to participate in the community as long as desired. All settings are situated within the same twenty-six-acre campus, sharing common social spaces, outdoor areas, and support services, which is intended to enhance familiarity and sustain social networks among staff members, people with dementia, and their caregivers.

Aging in place within a long-term care facility

Aging in place can refer to long-term settings designed to accommodate residents within the same environment throughout various stages of the disease. These long-term care settings use design, as well as other strategies, to differentiate between residents at various stages of the disease.

For example, the Friendship House of the Cedar Lake Home Campus in West

Figure 3.2

Repetitive household modules allow grouping based on functional ability and ease residents' transition between units. (First Floor, Friendship House, Cedar Lake Home Campus, West Bend, Wisconsin)

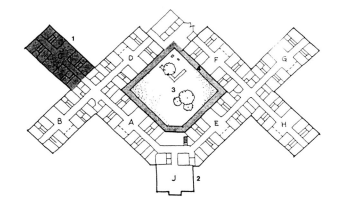

Figure 3.3

The three similar residential modules are connected by a common, public space. The modulation allows internal transfers based on changing abilities and needs. (Woodside Place, Oakmont, Pennsylvania; drawing by David Hoglund.)

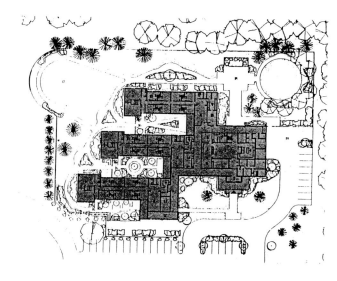

Figure 3.4

Two residential modules (*bottom*) offer spaces to accommodate a wide range of activities for more independent residents, while two modules (*top*) are designed for a high level of dependency. All modules are located under one roof and are served by the same staff. (Namesté, Colorado Springs, Colorado)

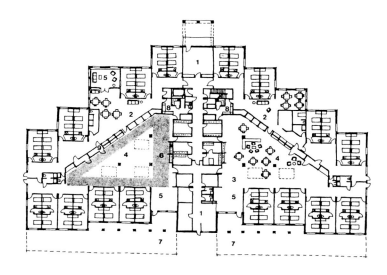

Bend, Wisconsin, was designed as a residential facility for 128 residents; the building comprises eight identical units, each of which houses 16 residents (fig. 3.2). The eight residential modules or "households" allow flexible grouping of residents according to level of abilities or other relevant criteria. This plan organization allows for within-building moves due to changing needs. The familiarity of the basic household to all residents limits confusion and disorientation after relocation to a strange environment.

Woodside Place in Oakmont, Pennsylvania, also employs repetitive household modules, each of which houses twelve residents, grouped according to level of AD (fig. 3.3). Because residents participate in activities in public spaces spaced throughout the facility, each unit is differentiated by color, signage, and decorative motifs to minimize confusion among residents in locating their own households. At the same time, sufficient consistency among units exists to offset disorientation after transfer.

Namesté, in Colorado Springs, Colorado, is a long-term care facility composed of four nonidentical household units designed to accommodate residents at differing levels of functional ability (fig. 3.4). High-functioning residents are housed in modules that accommodate a great deal of activity and social interaction, while low-functioning residents occupy households without such spaces, in the belief that these would be underutilized by this population. However, such a belief may be self-fulfilling, as low-functioning residents may experience insufficient stimulation in these households, further promoting their decline in functional ability and social skills. Obviously, such an issue involves critical placement and programming decisions, as well as architectural strategies.

Toward the Deinstitutionalization of Care Environments

Because people with dementia do not require extensive medical intervention, particularly in the earlier stages of the disease, the institutional or "medical model" of the hospital or health care facility is often deemed inappropriate for the design and operation of environments for people with dementia. This model was common to most nursing homes and other long-term care facilities in the past, and many facilities continue to adopt this institutional inheritance in terms of both design and management for lack of careful consideration of alternatives or through the absence of a better prototype.

Increasingly, the model of the home or residential setting has been substituted as a more humane, potentially more cost effective, and more therapeutic alternative to the institutional model. The creation of a "homelike" environment is a primary strategy for deinstitutionalization. Operationalization of this concept varies among facilities and facility types; however, it is typically limited to few and minor applications, such as allowing residents to bring a piece of furniture from home to the facility. Research has identified several basic categories of design applications toward deinstitutionalization: (1) external imagery, (2) internal imagery, (3) the incorporation of familiar activity spaces, and (4) organizational solutions.

Imagery is an important tool for promoting noninstitutionalization, with both exterior and interior imagery playing a key role. Many of the facilities examined—particularly newly constructed facilities—adopted a noninstitutional, residentially inspired exterior design, manipulating large buildings into small-scale elements and avoiding monolithic structures, materials, and forms.

Cedar Acres Adult Day Center in Janesville, Wisconsin, is an ideal example of residential exterior imagery (fig. 3.5). In fact, this day care center for twenty-four clients is located in a 100-year-old farmhouse set on seven sprawling acres of natural land. Although a major addition to the home was made to accommodate its new occupants, the center maintains its picturesque, domestic appearance and ambience, perhaps its greatest attraction.

Noninstitutional external imagery was also achieved on a larger scale at Woodside Place in Oakmont, Pennsylvania (fig. 3.6). This long-term care facility is designed to accommodate three "houses" of twelve residents each; the sloped roof pattern and arrangement of the houses sets each house apart and emphasizes the small scale of these units rather than the large scale of the total building. In addition, the scale of plantings and the window treatments and exterior finishes reinforce this domestic imagery.

Figure 3.5
Participating in day care activities in this nineteenth century farmhouse gives one the feeling of a pleasant outing in the country. (Cedar Acres Adult Day Center, Janesville, Wisconsin)

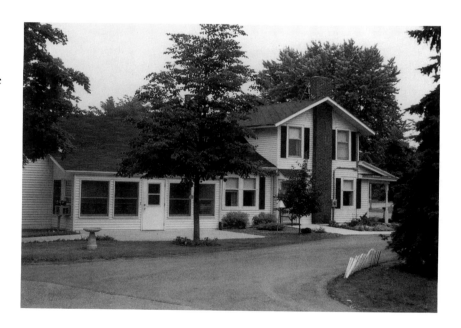

Internal imagery

Even greater attention has been paid to utilizing noninstitutional imagery in the interior environment of most facilities. Domestic and residential appearance has been enhanced through the use of noninstitutional finishes and furnishings, such as wood for hand railings, carpeting on the floors, fabric upholstery (Scotchgarded for protection) on sofas and chairs, and domestic wallpapers, furnishings, curtains, and bedcovers in residents' rooms. Many

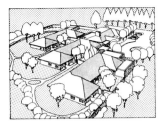

Figure 3.6
The pitched roofs and house form of each residential module deemphasize the large scale of the thirty-six-resident building. (Woodside Place, Oakmont, Pennsylvania; drawing by David Hoglund.)

Figure 3.7
Wesley Hall in Chelsea, Michigan, was a pioneering experiment in renovating an institutional environment into a more residential-looking setting. This illustration demonstrates "deinstitutionalization" through the use of domestic furnishings and interior finishes. (Wesley Hall, Chelsea, Michigan)

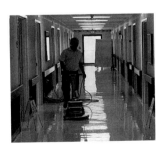

Figure 3.8
Stereotypical "institutional" corridor.

facilities exhibited artwork depicting significant local scenes or events. Others emphasized the domestic nature of public spaces such as kitchens, back porches, living rooms, and bedrooms through familiar, residential decoration, furnishings, and appliances. Perhaps the greatest commonality shared by the facilities examined in this document is their consistent effort—to varying extents—to emphasize noninstitutional imagery in their interior environment (fig. 3.7).

Two particular design features are commonly associated with the interior imagery of the institutional environment: long, double-loaded corridors (fig. 3.8), and the formal nurses' station. These features can easily incorporate noninstitutional design alternatives.

Elimination of Institutional Corridors

One particular, important strategy for enhancing noninstitutional ambience is the elimination of traditional, long, "institutional" corridors. The double-loaded corridors of resident's rooms were shortened, modified, or completely eliminated in many of the facilities examined. The Corinne Dolan Alzheimer

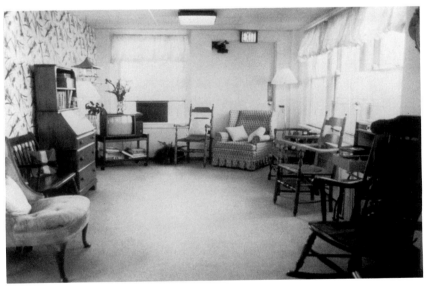

Center in Chardon, Ohio, is an example of a facility without a formal corridor (fig. 3.9). In this residential care facility, resident's rooms open directly onto a large, common activity area, ringed with a wandering path differentiated from the activity core by floor texture and color. Residents negotiate the transition from room to wandering path to activity area without the need for any corridors at all. At the same time, staff and resident visibility to this primary activity area is greatly enhanced, ensuring both orientation and safety and security (thereby avoiding the common complaint about short, disjointed corridors as disorienting to residents and detrimental to staff surveillance).

Figure 3.9
The central activity area is surrounded by residents' rooms. This strategy completely eliminates the conventional corridor. (Corinne Dolan Alzheimer Center, Chardon, Ohio)

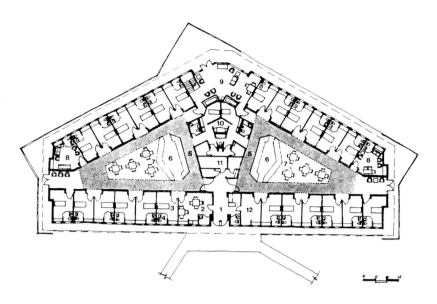

Deemphasis of the Nurses' Station

The traditional, fortress-like nursing station, often mandated by state nursing home codes, is frequently perceived as an icon of the institutional environment. Unfortunately, its use is not solely restricted to conventional nursing homes, as the nursing station appears in modified form in many supposedly noninstitutional settings, such as group homes. When the nursing station is disguised, eliminated, or somehow domesticated, the noninstitutional nature of the environment can be greatly enhanced. New Perspective Group Home #4 in Mequon, Wisconsin, adopted such a strategy. In this group home for twelve residents, the nursing station was replaced by the kitchen counter, over which staff members can observe residents in the great room, kitchen and dining area, and enclosed inner courtyard (fig. 3.10). A small desk in a corner of the activity room is used for charting and paperwork, but the owner discourages staff members from storing any materials in this area. Because of its isolation from the locus of activities, staff members utilize this space only occasionally for specific tasks that require concentration or privacy. (The design of New Perspective also utilizes the massing of its attached, auxiliary apartment to reinforce the residential, exterior image of the facility.)

Residential activities and activity spaces

A noninstitutional ambience and environment can also be enhanced through the incorporation of domestic activities and activity spaces into the facility. Participation in activities such as food preparation, laundry folding, "babysitting" with local children, and light housekeeping may have a positive therapeutic effect for residents, and residential spaces designed to accommodate these activities will also reinforce domestic atmosphere and operation.

Elderkare in Beloit, Wisconsin, is a newly designed group home for twelve residents that incorporates several such domestic activity areas. Residents par-

Figure 3.10
The kitchen in this group home is also a center for unobtrusive control and a locus for group activities. (New Perspective Group Home #4, Mequon, Wisconsin)

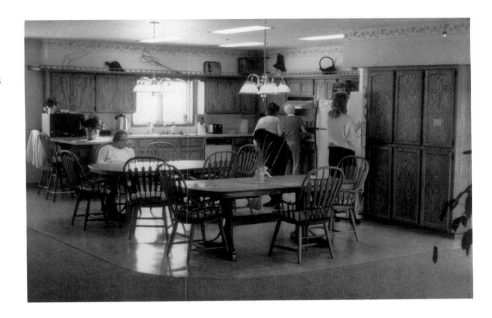

ticipate in social and therapeutic activities in the homelike kitchen, the living/ dining room and family lounge, and a small, corner laundry room. These spaces resemble their domestic counterparts in both physical appearance and function, reinforcing the sense of "home" in the facility among residents. (In addition, this facility was designed to include a typical, residential two-car garage, important as much for its reinforcement of domestic imagery as for its functional usage.)

Organizational solutions

Deemphasis of the institutional environment can take place not only in a physical sense, but also through manipulation of social and management aspects of the facility. Several examples illustrate this approach.

"Noninstitutional" Staff Background

An important organizational policy to combat "institutional" management and staff behavior was also identified during the case study visits. Several facilities indicated that hiring preferences dictated staff members without a previous background in nursing home work or care for people with dementia. Such past experience may be perceived as a potential negative and institutional influence on staff members, who may carry over preconceptions about long-term care and people with dementia into the new facility. A preference for staff without a nursing home background was particularly noticeable in nontraditional setting types such as group and boarding homes (see under "Staffing issues").

Capitalizing on Strengths and Limitations

Staff members' individual strengths can also be utilized to reinforce a non-institutional atmosphere. In several care facilities in Honolulu, Hawaii, newly arrived employees from the Philippines without a great deal of education are hired to help with housekeeping and meal preparation activities. Although they frequently cannot communicate with day care participants due to language differences, these staff members make a significant contribution to the participants' quality of life by working together with them in these familiar household activities. Many residents would rather fold linen than listen to "current events" in reality orientation; at the same time, these staff members pride themselves on sharing in the "care" of the participants in this fashion.

Cost Issues

Cost issues related to the construction and operation of a facility for people with dementia often are a primary concern for family members, as well as facility developers, planners, and administrators. Facilities frequently described their own financial situation (both positive and negative) as unique: however, many common problems and solutions arose in the course of these case studies. Frequently, a tactic adopted by one facility in a particular condition might be fruitfully adopted by others in a similar situation. These insights, though somewhat superficial, may give rise to creative strategies for the resolution of cost issues for other facility administrators, planners, and designers.

Determinants of feasibility

Economic feasibility depends on many factors that may make an identical project economically feasible or even profitable in one area and unfeasible in another. Such factors include the interest rates on loans; the cost of land in a particular neighborhood, city, or region; the restrictive or unrestricted nature of local regulatory codes; the selection of an urban versus a rural location; and local norms regarding staff salaries. Although these issues are not discussed further here, one must recognize that all are critical variants in determining the cost of construction and of care, making unadjusted, lateral comparison of construction costs and service charges between facilities very difficult.

All else being equal, a major issue in determining economic feasibility is the question of the ideal size of the resident population. Day care centers in particular wrestle with the question of the appropriate number of clients to achieve economic feasibility. Many administrators of day care facilities noted that day care at the scale usually recommended from a therapeutic perspective (fewer than twenty participants) is difficult to provide from an economic standpoint. Financial support of some type or membership in a continuum of care campus that absorbs some of their operating costs is almost always necessary to maintain a center at this census level. Increasingly, day care providers are examining the possibility of raising the number of participants to at least thirty to achieve independent economic feasibility, a fact that has significant design implications. A potential design strategy for day care centers serving over thirty residents simultaneously involves subdivision of residents and spaces into small households, similar to those often adopted in long-term care facilities. This scheme controls the scale of the environment and the amount of stimulation with which a client is faced.

*Payment based on
level of care provided*

A relatively innovative concept for determining charges for care for people with dementia was mentioned during case study visits to two independent facilities. Facilities adopting this strategy assess the charge to an individual resident based on the specific level of care that he or she requires, according to the individual's needs as determined from an objective checklist of services and levels of functional ability (developed by the facility). For example, residents who are incontinent, are not ambulatory, or wander pay more for their care in a boarding or group home than do other residents under the assumption that caring for residents with these characteristics is more expensive in terms of staff time and wear on surfaces, materials, and furnishings. The idea that residents should bear the cost of serving their individual needs is not an entirely new idea: most facilities already assess individual charges for "special" services not shared by all residents, such as transportation or beauty shop visits. However, such a fee structure has not often been extended to include other, more "care"-related services, such as a need for greater assistance with toileting, eating, or other activities of daily living.

Elderkare, a for-profit group home in Beloit, Wisconsin, is a facility structured on the concept of payment per level of care. Residents in the facility are assessed at admission according to a fourteen-point checklist developed by facility administrators and are reassessed every six months (or more frequently if required). The facility director noted that this strategy of assessment appears perfectly reasonable to most family members, who are accustomed to retail market or even health care charges assessed according to the products or services received. It is only among long-term care providers that this strategy seems innovative or foreign. At Elderkare, assessment based on level of care required automatically ensures that, as residents progress through the stages of the disease, funds are immediately available to pay for the increased staff time that such a population demands. In addition, this strategy may affect a facility's policy regarding acceptance of residents who may require additional care and supervision. According to the "traditional," equitable assessment strategy, it is in the best interest of the facility to attract residents in the early stages of the disease who require less care, as a more advanced population would require more expensive care without consequent additional reimbursement. With the pay-per-level-of-care strategy, facilities may be less reluctant to admit stage 2 and 3 residents or to take on those residents who may rapidly progress to these stages.

One day care provider also mentioned that this strategy may be adopted in their center to assess more fairly one or two participants who are currently receiving expensive skilled nursing care during their time at the center—a cost that has been unfairly borne by all participants until now. Other care providers suggest that this strategy may be unethical and needless. As all participants/residents will eventually require intensive care, they are not "unfairly" assessed when they pay a small amount extra to help to offset the cost of caring for participants in advanced stages, thereby helping to maintain care that is affordable for all family caregivers.

Because the Alois Alzheimer Center was designed to provide a continuum of care, a payment system was implemented based on a resident's level of care and staffing needs. Administrators felt that it was more ethical to charge less money for individuals who require less care, guidance, and supervision and to charge more for those who require more. Utilizing a modified Haycox Dementia Rating Scale, the individual is assessed and assigned by total score into a range of scores at each payment rate. The individual is reassessed on a quarterly basis at a care conference with family members, and the rate is adjusted depending upon the current level of care required. It is not unusual to experience a rate decrease, as individual functioning frequently improves, particularly after admission to the center.

Such an assessment strategy has implications for physical design as well as for staffing levels. The pay-per-level-of-care strategy generates increased income when low-functioning residents are admitted to a facility, income that can be used for environmentally therapeutic interventions as well as for increased staffing levels. Administrators considering the adoption of this assessment strategy must independently determine the best mix of residents (in terms of numbers, personalities, and functional abilities) and subsequent staffing levels for their facility and balance this equation with consideration of their own therapeutic goals, environmental intervention strategies, and the economic "best interests" of their population.

Cost for continuum of care membership

Several facility administrators noted that membership in a continuum of care campus or a formal organization of several facility types has its own special costs and benefits. For such facilities, balancing one's own budget and projecting resident costs depends not only upon the cost of providing care in that individual setting, but also on cost of other services and programs that must be shared by all member settings. For example, a group home that belongs to a continuum of care campus must account not only for the cost of providing care for its own residents, but also for a percentage of the cost of the campus-wide club house, park, swimming pool, and church; the salaries of the campus music therapist, research director, maintenance staff, minister, large administrative staff, and support group director; and the cost of maintaining a campus public relations department, research office, and other auxiliary services. Moreover, in a continuum of care arrangement, more profitable facilities frequently also help to support less profitable services and environments deemed important to the community.

Depending upon the strategy developed for billing each facility on the campus, membership in a continuum of care may result in higher costs and subsequently higher charges to residents than those at an independent facility. In addition, facilities in a continuum of care may be required financially to support services and specialty staff that are less than optimally useful to their own residents. Given the opportunity to invest funds independently on auxiliary staff and resources, facility directors may opt for choices different from those selected and provided for the entire campus. For example, a day care center without a research agenda and with other, more pressing needs might, given the option, choose to invest its "auxiliary resource" funds currently dedicated to the salary of a campus-wide research director into increasing its own full time staffing level or constructing a kitchenette in the activity room for the use of its clients.

On the other hand, because of their membership in a continuum of care, facilities may have access to many resources on campus that they may not have been able to afford independently and may not have been able to purchase for occasional use. For example, an independent group home may not be able to afford to purchase a van to transport its residents during local field trips. The prohibitive cost of renting a van for occasional use may force the staff to either restrict the residents to in-house activities or take only a few residents out at a time in staff members' cars, which may be impossible, depending on staffing levels in the facility. However, in New Perspective Group Home #4 in Mequon, Wisconsin, residents may soon have access to a van for field trips and transportation to appointments. New Perspective #4 is one of five community-based group homes owned and operated by the company, whose director is currently considering the purchase of a van for use by residents of the five homes. Because the cost of a van can be reasonably shared by the five settings, taking residents out for field trips may soon be both practical and affordable.

The location of a facility on a continuum of care campus may also offer residents access to nearby resources that might have been prohibitively distant from an independent facility. In addition, membership in a continuum of care may be a reasonable strategy to ensure the provision of less profitable but important therapeutic services and settings. Day care is frequently such a service—many day care centers might not exist if forced to operate on an independent budget.

"Down-licensing" as a strategy for cost containment

One complaint logged against traditional nursing homes as a setting for the care of people with dementia is that, because this population does not require intensive medical care until the end stages of the disease, environments for their use should not always be required to adopt expensive, "hospital" model construction. Regulatory requirements such as a central nurses' station and its spatial control implications are not only unnecessary for and underutilized by this population, but also frequently counterproductive from a therapeutic stance. One strategy for combating such "overconstruction" has been the growing trend to target and license facilities for people with dementia as boarding homes, community-based residential facilities, or facility types at other levels of licensing that do not require expensive nursing home-level construction. The Alzheimer Care Center in Gardiner, Maine, is one such facility. Its planners applied for special "boarding home" licensing for the facility, in part as a strategy for cost containment. This model project was partially funded by the state, and its planners intended to demonstrate that, by licensing and providing care at the level of a boarding rather than a nursing home, the state would save money in residential care for people with dementia. In reality, the cost of care at the center is only slightly lower than that of nursing homes in the area. Although money was saved on certain aspects of construction, additional money has been dedicated to maintaining higher-than-anticipated staffing levels required by the residents. However, the director of the facility feels that, although down-licensing in this instance did not function as a strategy to contain costs, money spent in the center is directed toward the actual needs of residents and not toward expensive, unnecessary overconstruction.

Residents and families of independent, unaffiliated boarding or rest homes may experience some difficulties with forced relocation, as residents who progress beyond the capabilities of the facility may be required to relocate more than once, a situation addressed by boarding home facilities that are situated on or affiliated with a broader continuum of care.

Comparison of square footage, amenities, and number of users

A basic calculation in projecting the construction cost of a planned facility is the multiplication of the total building's size (square footage) by the cost of construction per square foot. The following analysis provides comparative data related to the square footage of various facilities. These data can serve as a partial planning reference in projecting the size and cost of new facilities.

The analysis in table 3.1 is a very rough comparison of the case studies. The residential component typically—but not always—includes bathrooms and toilet rooms, depending on spatial organization.

Staffing Issues

Several issues related to staffing levels, positions, and spaces arose in the course of this research. While these issues vary in their degree of rootedness in the environment, they are nonetheless important considerations and present opportunities for facility planners and designers.

Preference for non–nursing home staff

In several facilities, a growing trend in the selection of staff members was noted; there seems to be a strong preference in many new facilities for staff members without previous experience in nursing homes or in the care of people with dementia. Woodside Place in Oakmont, Pennsylvania, is one such facility. The intention here is to staff the facility—a boarding home—with personnel who do not have previous negative impressions or biases about working with people with dementia, not uncommon among those with past work experiences in nursing homes, where people with dementia are often perceived as a difficult population and assignment to the special care unit for Alzheimer's disease may be considered an undesirable position. By hiring personnel without such past experiences, administrators at Woodside hope to instill a positive attitude toward working with people with dementia in their "care attendants" (not "nursing assistants," another nursing home convention). The Corinne Dolan Alzheimer Center in Chardon, Ohio, and the Alzheimer Care Center in Gardiner, Maine, both employ a similar philosophy. Administrators at the Alzheimer Care Center attribute their very high staff retention rate and morale at least in part to this factor. It is also reasonable (although not substantiated) to speculate that a correlation may exist between work condi-

Table 3.1 Comparative Analysis of Area to User Ratios in Selected Facilities

Facility	Size (square feet)		Total Area	Number of Users	Area (square feet) per User
	Residential Component	Activity and Public Spaces			
Group homes					
New Perspective	1,750	3,250	5,000	12	416
Helen Bader	5,488	11,112 (incl. ed. center)	16,600	24	666
Elderkare	3,000	2,200	5,200	12	433
Day care/respite care centers					
Hale Kako'O	1,700	1,000	2,700 (+1,800 for services)	12 respite 12.25 day	225 ~50
Cedar Acres	—	3,520	3,520 (+800 for offices)	average 21	167
Saint Ann	—	1,750	1,750	maximum 20	90
Long-term care facilities					
Alexian Village	13,900	5,600 (+3,000 for patio)	19,100	40	477
California Pacific	4,000	5,500 (incl. courtyard)	9,500	21	452
Corrine Dolan	5,400	8,600	14,000	24	583
Namesté	11,500	12,800	24,300	64	379
Woodside Place	6,800	16,200	23,000	36	638

tions and atmosphere (including the nature of the environment) and staff morale and retention.

The Cedar Lake Home Campus Friendship House in West Bend, Wisconsin, has—like many other facilities—developed its own, in-house training program for its nursing assistants to instill its care philosophy and a positive orientation toward working with people with dementia in its employees. Although the program runs at great cost to the facility, administrators believe that staff background has important implications for the quality of care of residents. (An additional reason for the development of an in-house training program may be the rural location of this facility, which may have difficulty attracting qualified employees. However, whether or not this is so, it does not negate the significance of the training program.)

Staff spaces: opposing philosophies concerning offices and retreats

There is some philosophical debate among facility administrators and owners about the proper role and use of designated spaces—both offices and "retreat" areas—for staff members. Some facility planners believe that staff members should spend all of their time with residents in the unit, including breaks and meals, to foster social interaction and a sense of community between staff and residents. These individuals often suggest that providing a separate, removed area for paperwork and/or staff retreat or relaxation encourages staff members to spend less time with residents. Other administrators believe that staff members require separate, private spaces for doing paperwork and administrative duties and that staff members benefit by spending time away from residents during breaks and meals. These two philosophies and the many examples that fall between have physical manifestations in the design and programming of facilities for people with dementia.

New Perspective Group Home #4 in Mequon, Wisconsin, represents a true example of the first philosophy: staff members are encouraged to spend all of their time with residents. In this facility, the activity room houses a small desk with no secure storage space, used by staff members for paperwork on an occasional basis. This is the only designated "staff space" in the facility; staff members share all meals, breaks, and other activities with residents. The owner of the facility believes that providing a large, private workspace or office encourages staff members to spend too much time on paperwork; this represents time away from the residents. However, because this group home is part of a larger network of group homes, it is logical to assume that this strategy is effective here because the paperwork load is relatively light and administrative duties are performed off-site in a central office. In addition, the relatively high functional level of residents permits them to accrue positive benefits from this "extra" time spent socializing with staff members.

In most facilities that assume a similar position, the conventional "nurses' station" is typically merged into a domestic kitchen, which provides a place for central observation, a work surface, and storage cabinets for necessary administrative materials.

Total access has its limitations. The Alois Alzheimer Center initially attempted to establish nontraditional, less formal stations or areas for nurses and staff to sit and work. In time, it was necessary to alter this plan, as it became increasingly clear that the open environment created conflicts: residents seeking attention would wander into these areas, taking things and constantly interrupting staff.

The Friendship House of Cedar Lake Home Campus represents the exclusive retreat philosophy. Here, both a staff lounge and a cafeteria for staff members from the eight resident households were deemed absolutely necessary. Administrators explained this need by pointing to the declining functional level of the population of this facility, almost all of whom now require skilled nursing care (not true when the facility first opened). Staff members perform intensive jobs similar to those in skilled nursing care facilities; they require a staff retreat area away from the residents for occasional breaks from the demands of the job. A separate staff cafeteria is also provided; staff members do not eat with residents, as most residents require constant assistance with eating. Furthermore, administrators report that, as most residents can no longer benefit from social interaction, allowing staff members to socialize on their breaks away from the unit does not represent a lost opportunity for residents. Even when residents maintain a high level of functioning, a separate space for a lunch break away from residents may have positive, revitalizing effects on staff members. It seems that the question of whether to provide a separate staff retreat area away from residents depends to a great degree on both the number and the functional level of residents. Of course, this is also tied to the legal issue of mandatory employee breaks, according to which a certain number and duration of rest periods are required by law.

Elderkare in Beloit, Wisconsin, falls between these two examples. Staff members here required a private space away from residents for office paperwork and administrative duties; the original office was constantly besieged by residents, leading to a decision to move the office into a former linen closet, hardly ideal for this purpose. However, staff members make a concerted effort to conduct as much "business" as possible while still interacting with residents. In fact, all staff meetings are intentionally held in the common area of the facility, "right in the middle of everything." Residents are permitted to participate in or observe these sessions. (The actual value of this participation is questionable.)

Administrators at the Alzheimer Care Center also found that the staff desk used by the facility nurse and social worker was overly accessible to rummaging and interruption by residents. This desk was moved from its original location in the middle of a wide corridor to a room that formerly served as a staff lounge. However, residents are permitted and even encouraged to wander freely and visit with staff members in the administrative office area, where staff work is not as sensitive to interruption.

The office of the activity director in one case study was a frequent stopping place for wandering residents. The director was not disturbed by the visits: during meetings and important calls, she simply closed the door to allow some privacy.

The auxiliary apartment as a device to improve quality of care

Two of the facilities examined include an auxiliary apartment occupied by a staff member. In both instances, the staff member receives free lodging in exchange for a willingness to be "on call" during the third shift, when only one aide is on duty. The addition of an auxiliary apartment supports many unique opportunities in these facilities.

At New Perspective Group Home #4, an attached apartment has a direct entrance to the facility from indoors, as well as a private, outdoor entrance (fig.

Figure 3.11

This auxiliary apartment
(9) has a direct entrance
to the facility from in-
doors. In addition to in-
creasing the effective
night staffing ratio, the addition of this auxiliary
apartment increases the
ease of keeping a facility
dog. (New Perspective
Group Home #4, Me-
quon, Wisconsin)

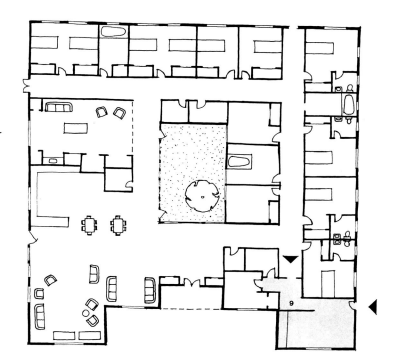

3.11). To assist the aide on duty, the staff member in the auxiliary apartment is summoned when the call button is pressed in any of the residents' rooms. Thus, the addition of a staff apartment saves management the cost of hiring two additional nighttime employees, one for each group home. The auxiliary apartment also provides an ideal residence for the facility dog, who belongs to the staff member residing in the apartment. This staff member assumes responsibility for the dog's care (often a problem in facilities with pets, as no one staff member oversees the needs of the pet), and the dog can easily be returned to the apartment when residents are agitated or overstimulated. Finally, the auxiliary apartment is a positive residential addition to the exterior of the facility, in both design and scale.

Minna Murra Lodge in Queensland, Australia, also provides an auxiliary apartment, occupied by its supervisor. In addition to the benefits of nighttime assistance that are afforded by this arrangement, the social spaces of the auxiliary apartment seem to double-function as an area for staff retreat and meetings. By night, they resume their function as the private apartment of the facility supervisor. The auxiliary apartment serves as one example of the use of the environment to gain other resources for the facility.

Auxiliary apartments often include a garage or private yard, truly residential features in the United States. In this way, the auxiliary apartment offers an architectural opportunity for enhancing a noninstitutional image.

The Right Location: Urban versus Rural Settings

More often than not, environments for people with dementia are planned and designed with a predetermined location in mind; this is particularly true of small-scale projects. The location may be a vacant basement of a church, a

Figure 3.12

Elderkare, a community-based group home, was built in a newly developing residential area in Beloit, Wisconsin. The site was selected primarily for the low cost of land in this neighborhood. In part because of the relatively low cost of the land, sufficient funds existed for the construction of a large (given its population) facility with private rooms for all residents, many small activity spaces, and a residential-looking two car garage. (Elderkare, Beloit, Wisconsin)

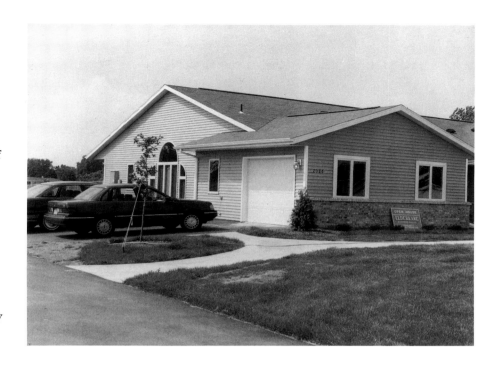

piece of land donated to a nonprofit group, or the corner of an existing facility. However, when the opportunity to choose a location for a new facility presented itself, many facility planners consciously considered the advantages and disadvantages of the extreme possibilities of rural and urban sites, as well as of the many alternatives in between. Furthermore, in numerous case studies where the site of the facility *was* predetermined, directors actively exploited the opportunities inherent in the location while minimizing weaknesses through good planning. Finally, those facilities that acquired a site through donation represent a third justification for consideration of this issue: in some instances, the donation of a building to a nonprofit, dementia care organization may be best leveraged through its sale to purchase a more appropriate site or building. Location is a key issue to be discussed when making such a decision.

The following is a list of many generalized positive and negative characteristics of rural and urban sites.

Rural setting

- Land cost may be relatively low. Therefore, a facility may be able to afford more land and may plan a larger, less restricted building form and more usable outdoor space than at a comparable urban site (fig. 3.12).
- The external image is often quite unrestricted by zoning regulations.
- Opportunities for access to natural landscape and ambience are frequently heightened.
- It may be difficult for employees, volunteers, and visitors (especially frail, single, elderly spouses) to reach the site if adequate public transportation does not exist. In addition, the pool of potential employees, volunteers, and

residents within the immediate area may be quite small, forcing the facility to draw residents and staff from a wide area.

- In the case of day care, provision of transportation for clients is often almost mandatory, given the distance of many clients from the facility, and the lack of adequate public transportation.

Urban setting

- Urban sites are frequently more accessible for employees, volunteers, and visitors than are rural sites. The pool of potential employees, volunteers, and residents in the immediate area is usually quite large.
- In general, land cost is high (as compared to rural settings), and, subsequently, sites are frequently small, outdoor space is limited, and building form is strictly dictated by the site.
- Urban environments often provide a great deal of stimulation in the outdoor environment, which can have positive or negative implications, depending on the resident population, the specific site conditions, and the source of stimulation.
- Community resources can frequently be found nearby.
- In the case of day care, there may be less need to provide transportation for clients in urban than in rural locations (although this was described as an important service by day care providers in both locations).

For example, the Helen Bader Center of the Milwaukee Jewish Home is located in a continuum of care campus on an urban site not far from downtown Milwaukee. In part because of its urban location, the center can depend upon a constant dedicated staff of full-time volunteers, drawn from the Jewish community of Milwaukee.

Suburban and small town locations fall somewhere between these two extremes. In many ways, the attributes of rural locations also apply to suburban sites, given the same tendency toward low-cost land and possible access to "picturesque" (if not rural) landscape. However, one important exception may exist; greater resistance to the development of a facility for people with dementia may be encountered in suburban residential communities than in either urban or rural neighborhoods. This may be due to both the frequently close proximity of the facility to its neighbors (unlike many rural sites) and the homogeneity of the existing population (unlike many urban sites). Of course, this is a generalization, and specific instances may vary widely.

Activity Areas

Activity spaces and communal areas represent the physical domain that manifests the most visible transformation in the recent history of facilities for people with dementia. The transition from "standard" facilities—comprising resident rooms, corridors, and a day room that doubles as a dining area—to "contemporary" facilities, with varied activity and public spaces, is both a qualitative and a quantitative change.

Spaces for large and small group activities frequently form the organizational core—literally the "living rooms"—of facilities for people with dementia.

Likewise, activity planning frequently represents the major thrust of therapeutic programming for this population. Because of their significance in the lives of residents, activities and spaces that accommodate them warrant careful analysis.

The physical and spatial organization of activity spaces

The wide variations found in the sample of case studies defy a generic typology of spatial organization. However, to organize the following discussion of the features and spatial attributes of activity spaces, a simple typology is offered. The two primary types of organizational schemes are (1) facilities with unified, central, large activity cores and (2) facilities with several dispersed, small activity spaces.

Unified, Central, Large Activity Cores.

This version of the central activity core model, with variations, is represented by several facilities, such as the Weiss Center in Philadelphia, Pennsylvania (fig. 3.13), and Namesté Alzheimer Center in Colorado Springs, Colorado.

A slightly different spatial representation of the central activity core model occurs in several facilities, in which activity areas are clustered physically in the core, but each area has a separate identity and clear boundaries exist between each activity space and its neighbors (fig. 3.14). The activity spaces have territorial affiliation with a particular residential module or household.

Several Dispersed, Small Activity Spaces

The Friendship House in West Bend, Wisconsin, is an example of a facility organized with many activity areas dispersed throughout the building. The dining room and kitchen and the adjoining living room are an integral part of each of the eight residential modules. In addition, the facility has a large dining/day room and a public entry lobby/living room on the ground floor. The "dispersed" model also has countless physical variations.

Several general qualities are associated with each type of organization.

Unified Central Core of Activity Areas
- Activities are directly accessible to all residents.
- Unobtrusive surveillance of activity areas is easy to maintain.
- Large activity spaces may be institutional in scale.
- Noise and stimulation levels may be high.
- Some variations partially or completely eliminate institutional corridors, although the substitution may be an equally nonresidential juxtaposition of public and private spaces.

Dispersed Activity Areas
- Great variety in ambience and locational choices for activities is provided.
- Potentially, a high degree of control of level of stimulation and noise is possible.

Figure 3.13

An example of a facility with a central activity core: all rooms face a common public space that includes a dining area, a defined gazebo, and an open zone for multipurpose activities. (Weiss Institute, Philadelphia Geriatric Center, Philadelphia, Pennsylvania)

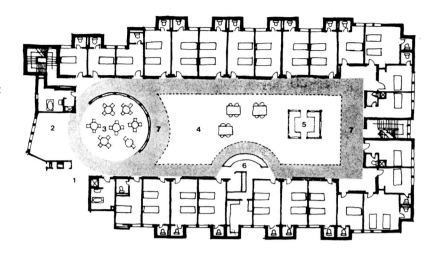

Figure 3.14

A variation of the "centralized activity space" model: four residential clusters surround activity spaces, including a protected central courtyard, two dens with patios, a dining room, and a living room. (Stonefield Home, Middleton, Wisconsin)

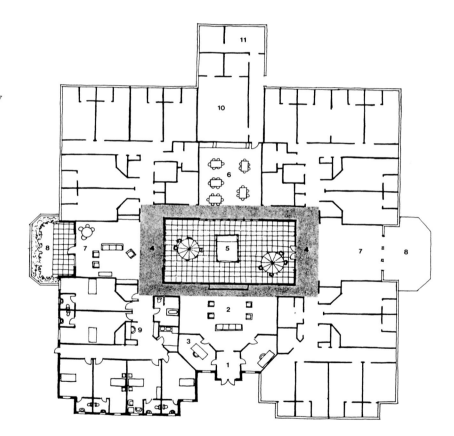

- The ease of separating an agitated resident from the rest of the group is increased.
- Domestic scale is maintained.
- Spaces are amenable to flexible scheduling.
- Unobtrusive surveillance of all spaces simultaneously may be difficult or impossible.

The Corinne Dolan Alzheimer Center represents a mixed model: it includes dispersed activity spaces such as a craft room, family rooms, and a living room, as well as the central dining and kitchen area for food-related activities.

Variety in activities and spaces

Case study visits vividly demonstrate that activities need not be limited to a few "conventional" offerings such as arts and crafts, music, and bingo. Many facilities, after considering the personalities, interests, and backgrounds of their own resident population, muster local resources and staff expertise to engage residents in such activities as taffy pulling, snow man construction, ice cream making, and trips to local cider mills, historic spots, and restaurants. In the same manner, activity spaces need not be limited to typical, institutional spaces such as day rooms or large activity areas that double function for dining. Music rooms, crafts lounges, general stores, kitchens, and indoor atria are examples of the types of spaces that can be created to offer variety and to support various types and levels of activity in environments for people with dementia. Variety can be beneficial for residents, who may enjoy participating in and observing many different activities and using varied spaces, even when these experiences are soon forgotten. Variety can also be beneficial for staff members, who may experience heightened enthusiasm and interest in varied activities and spaces, as well as for family members, who may feel more positive toward the care environment and their family member when he or she is having fun engaged in varied and interesting activities and spaces.

Tapping Local Resources

One means of increasing the variety of activities and activity spaces available to a facility is the rigorous pursuit of appropriate local services and citizens to complement a facility's own activities and personnel resources. For example, the Milwaukee Jewish Home in Milwaukee, Wisconsin, is located on a continuum of care campus that includes special features such as a delicatessen restaurant for occasional outings and a synagogue used by residents for weekly services. Facilities might create their own such resources by scheduling a local beautician, podiatrist, massage therapist, or minister and local musical entertainment during unconventional hours. Additional local resources that can be utilized by one or more facilities for people with dementia, on alternate days, include a local high school pool, movie theater, restaurant, and bowling alley. Even the nearby shopping center might serve as an excellent location for walking and window shopping with residents before it opens for business in the morning and during off-hours.

Volunteers from the community are another local resource that can enrich the activity program in environments for people with dementia. For example, a local minister can be enlisted to lead weekly religious services in the facility, in a quiet room converted each week for this purpose. Local people may be engaged to lead classes on ceramics, to talk about local history, and to offer theatrical entertainment.

Maintaining a Homelike, Familiar Domestic Ambience

Activities and activity spaces frequently play a significant role in establishing the atmosphere of a facility, particularly in those facilities that maintain a residential, noninstitutional ambience. Various familiar, domestic activities, such as gardening, washing dishes, folding laundry, dusting and polishing, making coffee, and sorting clothes, are usually manageable activities for the person with dementia, even into advanced stages of the disease. Such activities have typically been performed throughout most individuals' lives: they are familiar and memorable, and do not require new learning. The incorporation of these activities and the spaces that support them—such as laundry rooms, gardening beds, accessible kitchens, and "woodshops"—reinforces the residential, noninstitutional nature of facilities for people with dementia, positively influencing staff and resident behavior.

The incorporation of household-related work into the program of activities should realistically be viewed as a therapeutic—and not necessarily a labor-saving—strategy. Aside from union concerns that residents may replace paid employees, residents performing household tasks do not actually replace regular staff members in maintenance and food preparation positions. In addition, any resident performing "jobs" around a facility must be paid for the work. Household jobs will typically take longer for the resident to accomplish than the staff member, will require staff supervision in many instances, and frequently must be "redone" by the staff member (at least in the case of dish washing and cleaning) to meet health and sanitation codes. However, the therapeutic benefits of heightened self-esteem, independence, and involvement in activities that are possible through the delegation of tasks to residents is certainly sufficient justification for allowing residents to participate in household activities.

Implications of the number of caregivers on activities and activity spaces

There is a strong and significant relationship between the number of caregivers in a setting and the number and nature of activities and activity spaces that can reasonably be accommodated. Many specific activity spaces (e.g., a small laundry room used for folding clothes with low-functioning residents) are only truly usable when there is sufficient staff and a sufficiently high staffing ratio to spare one staff member for this small group or one-on-one activity. Likewise, kitchenettes, crafts lounges, and beauty shops will all receive more use by residents when staffing levels accommodate these activities. Elderkare, a group home in Beloit, Wisconsin, employs a 1:4 staffing ratio of direct care employees to residents. This strategy allows staff members to individually supervise one or two residents cooking in the kitchen, folding laundry in the laundry room, or engaged in grooming activities in the powder room, while large group activities occupy the majority of the residents. Although such advice may appear self-evident, it should be taken as a warning against over-expenditure for the creation of sophisticated, isolated, single-purpose activity areas that require staff surveillance for use at the expense of an adequate staffing budget to allow the use of such spaces. Such a principle also suggests that, when possible, activity areas should be designed to allow maximum use by residents with or without constant supervision.

"Resource-rich" environments

Regardless of the functional level of residents or day care clients, an environment that is relatively poor in resources or "things to do" will deprive its residents of most opportunities for unprogrammed, informal, and individual activities. A resource-rich environment—including household items for dusting, sorting, and discussing; textured items to touch; craft items to manipulate; musical instruments or a radio to play; pets to watch or with which to play, etc.—is necessary to accommodate unstructured activities at all levels of functioning. There is little that even potentially active and engaged residents can do independently in a sterile, institutional environment deprived of objects to which residents have ready access. In such a setting, residents are forced to rely solely on large-group, programmed activities to occupy and entertain themselves.

The relation of activities to functional level

Facilities for people with dementia are constantly confronted with the dilemma of how to relate activity programming and spaces to stages of the disease and functional levels. Activities should challenge and stimulate residents to maintain their highest possible level of functioning, but many large-group activities seeking to strike an appropriate balance may actually be boring for some residents and frustrating for others. At the same time, facilities are loathe to neglect either group by gearing activities toward one end of the scale or the other. This issue can be partially addressed by providing simultaneously a variety of activities—large- and small-group and independent activities geared toward varying functional levels. The Corinne Dolan Alzheimer Center provides four program options of various types of activities to meet the needs of residents at various stages of functional ability and those with various interests. In addition to one program that emphasizes traditionally "masculine" activities such as yard work, maintenance projects, and sports, the Corinne Dolan Alzheimer Center offers three levels of programs that range from high intensity (e.g., structured social activities such as discussion groups, crafts, and lifelong learning classes for residents who can communicate verbally, sustain focus and attention, and cooperate with others) to moderate intensity, structured around home activities (e.g., gardening, laundry, shop work, and housekeeping), to a flexibly structured, low-intensity program (e.g., music groups, parties, simple games, and individual discussions and projects).

Many facilities provide varied activity spaces to accommodate simultaneous activities by residents at different functional levels (or with varying personalities and preferences). Activity spaces may differ in size; location; level of visual, aural, and olfactory stimulation; and type of equipment provided. Examples of such spaces include the family lounge, front porch, music corner, kitchenette, great room, exercise room, craft niche, screened back patio, indoor atrium, and smoking room.

A strategy of separation is often adopted in the belief that high-functioning residents have little tolerance for those at a lower functional level and that prolonged contact between these groups may frustrate and produce negative consequences for both. Many activity directors, however, are reluctant to "skim" all high-functioning residents into separate activities and activity spaces, as this group serves as a positive role model for low functioning residents. One possible resolution of this dilemma involves strategies that offer varying types of experiences for residents at different functional levels. For example, playing with clay can be a creative and challenging opportunity for self-expression for high-functioning residents and a purely tactile and sensory experience for low-functioning residents. Bumper bowling is another example of an activity that allows residents to participate with varying levels of motor skills. In this version of the game, inflatable "bumpers" are placed in the gutters of the bowling alley, which will not affect the game of high-functioning residents but will guarantee success among residents with deteriorated motor skills. The principle of graded challenge can also be applied to develop activities that allow all residents to participate at their own levels, with different kinds of success for each. For example, "gerobic" exercise classes can be designed for residents to participate fully, participate to a limited extent while seated in a chair, clap along to the music to accompany exercising residents, and passively observe.

The relation of activities to time of day and day of week

The principle of "normalization" suggests that, as in "normal," domestic life, the type and location of activities and activity spaces should be related to the time of day and day of week. In ordinary, residential life, the type and location of activities are closely related to the time of day and the day of week: breakfast at 7:30 a.m. in the kitchen, nap between two and three p.m. in the bedroom, and lox and bagel and the *New York Times* in the sun room on Sunday morning. Familiar and habitual patterns are part of people's lives, including people with dementia. Facilities for people with dementia frequently make creative efforts to relate the type and location of activities to time of day and day of week. Such scheduling also considers residents' peak performance times for demanding activities and staff schedules and shift changes.

For example, many facilities schedule more activities—especially demanding activities—in the morning, when the level of concentration seems to be higher. Outdoor activities are scheduled in the morning in facilities where hot afternoon sun prohibits these later in the day. Mid-day activities often include food preparation for lunch or snacks, and afternoons consist of less demanding activities and rest periods. Activities are also frequently scheduled and located to keep residents busy and away from entrance areas during shift changes, as this activity is agitating for residents and may result in increased attempts to wander away from the facility. Evening events are frequently social in nature and attempt to limit the level of stimulation among residents prior to sleep.

In the same way, several facilities attempt to maintain those unique events that signify weekend versus weekday—for most people, the week does not normally continue undifferentiated. In particular, weekends are frequently associated with religious activities and social events. Solutions for tapping local resources suggested earlier represent a means of continuing this normal weekly pattern of activities. At the New Perspective Group Home #4 in Mequon, Wisconsin, Friday nights are always dedicated to a popular weekly dance held in the activity room. This social event maintains the normal pattern of weekend evening outings, which may be familiar to and anticipated by residents. Staff members at the Alzheimer Care Center in Gardiner, Maine, suggest that Saturdays in this home are normally utilized as a "day off" for both staff and residents. The relaxing pattern of Saturdays in most homes has been emulated, with mornings are devoted to leisure and individual activities and afternoons spent watching a movie or engaged in other relaxing activities. Many facilities have also adopted the normal and practical pattern of scheduling family and visitor activities for Sundays, a traditional "family" time.

The Appropriate Level of Sensory Stimulation

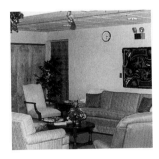

Figure 3.15
This day care center adopts a tranquil, restful, quiet, and calming decorating scheme in terms of colors, furnishings, wall hangings, and floor surfaces. (St. Ann Day Care Center, St. Francis, Wisconsin)

A debate continues among formal and informal caregivers and researchers regarding the appropriate amount and type of sensory stimulation for people with dementia. Hypotheses regarding the relationship between level of stimulation and residents' behavior frequently contradict each other. In simple terms, one position maintains that relatively high levels of physical, visual, aural, olfactory, and social stimulation are necessary to encourage activity and maintain function among people with dementia and that low levels of stimulation lead to null behavior and passivity. The opposing position argues that high levels of stimulation promote agitation, frustration, and confusion among people with dementia and that peaceful, tranquil, low stimulus settings are comforting and enhance concentration. In actuality, most facilities adopt a strategy that falls somewhere between these two extremes.

The most significant finding regarding this issue is the wide range of possible "appropriate" levels of stimulation. Staff members repeatedly stressed the great differences in preferred and tolerated stimulation among individual residents, which varied with personality, past life experiences, stage of the disease, time of day, and particular source of stimulation. Because of diversity in preferred levels of stimulation, it is important to create a physical and emotional environment that meets the needs of individuals in various stages of the disease process and to support a program based on the residents' level of functioning. This section recounts opinions and findings expressed in various facilities regarding four types of stimulation: (1) visual, (2) aural, (3) olfactory, and (4) social.

Visual stimulation

The literature on appropriate types and levels of visual stimulation is divided between approaches supporting the use of bright colors to counteract visual deficits and provide sufficient visual stimulation and those recommending soft, unobtrusive, "tranquil" colors and patterns to combat agitation and over-stimulation. Most facilities seemed to adopt the latter strategy (fig. 3.15). However, prevailing patterns do not confirm either position, and there seems to be little hard evidence in support of either at this time. This question certainly warrants further, conclusive research.

In addition to the question of color, there are other, less controversial sources of visual stimulation that were moderated in these facilities. Disturbing and distracting glare from direct sunlight was frequently reduced through window treatment and choice of materials and surfaces for tabletops and counter and floor surfaces. Decorating schemes for resident rooms were frequently selected as much to provide visual interest and variety as to aid identification by residents. Finally, outdoor areas were appreciated as much for the change of visual and other sensory stimulation they provide—even in the winter, when these spaces were not physically accessible—as for the variety of activities that can be supported outdoors.

Aural stimulation

Aural stimulation in particular seems to affect various residents in different ways. Administrators and staff members at the Alzheimer Care Center in Gardiner, Maine, planned and conducted a "quiet week" study to examine the effect of reducing noise and other stimulation levels in their facility for one week. During this time, the television volume was kept low, staff members spoke at moderated levels, and special efforts were directed at limiting sound from doorbells, alarms, beepers, and telephones. Although the results have not yet been reported, staff members found that reduced noise levels seemed to affect individual residents differently. Many residents seemed to miss the high level of stimulation, acting bored and restless. However, a few residents seemed to benefit greatly from the reduced noise level, displaying much less agitated behavior and greater concentration. Staff members now assert that preference for different levels of aural stimulation may vary significantly with personality and past job and life experiences. For example, a resident who had always worked in a demanding position requiring constant concentration and a very quiet work environment was among those residents who seemed to benefit most from reduced noise levels. There is a general agreement that particular loud and erratic sources of noise, such as doorbells, alarms, and telephones, are especially intrusive and disturbing to residents.

Ensuring variety and choice in possible levels of aural and other forms of stimulation frequently was adopted as a strategy to address the needs of a disparate resident population. Many facilities noted the need for a quiet room or a private space for use by agitated or overstimulated residents, although several residential facilities felt that this need was adequately addressed by resident rooms, especially in facilities with private rooms. Facilities also discussed the need to program both quiet and noisy activities and to offer choice among these.

Olfactory stimulation   Like aural stimulation, olfactory stimulation has both positive and negative forms. Facilities spent a great deal of effort and money on the control of unpleasant smells such as urine and strong cleaning product odors, which are irritating to residents, staff, and visitors and detract from the residential ambience of the facility. In fact, unattractive odors were not evidenced in any of the facilities visited, even given the higher-than-anticipated rate of incontinence reported in most settings. This was true of both those facilities with carpeted floors and fabric materials and surfaces and those with more typical (and institutional) vinyl surfaces. This fact would seem to negate the argument that residential-looking materials cannot be cleaned properly to control odor and so are inappropriate in facilities for people with dementia.

Facilities also discussed creative ways to utilize pleasant odors as an attractive source of stimulation for residents. Cooking odors in particular were perceived as a pleasant source of olfactory stimulation. Recognizing the strong link between sense of smell and memory, many facilities directed aromas of baking and cooking in the kitchen toward their dining areas, hoping that these smells would assist residents in remembering meal times and happy past associations with eating and food. Gardens and outdoor areas are another positive source of olfactory stimulation. Woodside Place, a long term care facility in Oakmont, Pennsylvania, intends to utilize different scents, including floral and pine, in the garden of each of its households as a pleasant source of stimulation for residents.

Social stimulation   An appropriate level of social stimulation refers to the type and amount of activity generated by interaction with or the co-presence of other persons that is therapeutic, desirable, or tolerable for the person with dementia.

Spatial Organization for Appropriate Social Stimulation

The two basic organizational models outlined under Activity Areas also differ in the amount of social stimulation they provide for residents in the two arrangements. Those who prefer settings designed around a large, common, open space used by all residents often subscribe to the belief that a critical number of residents is necessary for the generation of sufficient social stimulation and activity to combat null and passive resident behavior. Accordingly, these facilities frequently provide primarily high stimulus activity areas for residents' use.

Facilities designed according to the opposite strategy (that of small households and household-related spaces) often provide primarily small common spaces intended to be used by a limited number of ("household") residents. These facilities subscribe to the belief that, in addition to being more comfortable with and better able to remember others in a small, family-sized group, residents in small households are exposed to a limited number of people at any one time, which is less stimulating (and therefore less agitating and confusing) for them.

Entering and Exiting

Frequent entering and exiting of the facility by visitors, delivery personnel, or staff members is a particular source of stimulation noted to be especially distracting to residents. Such activity often interrupts residents' concentration and prompts them to attempt to exit the facility as well. Shift changes were noted as an especially critical time, when staff members are coming and going. Administrators mentioned that activities scheduled during this time were located away from the entrances to minimize distraction from this source. Staggering shift change hours also limited the amount of distraction from staff members conversing, packing and unpacking personal belongings, putting on and taking off coats in the winter, and opening and closing doors.

This issue was particularly relevant in day care centers, where coming and going is more intensive throughout the day. A common suggestion was to design the entrance and the coat storage areas so that these are not visible from the main activity areas. Facilities also attempted to address this problem when it arose after construction through the use of various visual buffers (e.g., light partitions, curtains, large planters).

More than one administrator mentioned that the number of observers, students, architects, and researchers interested in visiting their facility generated a constant flow of traffic that was distracting to residents. St. Ann Day Care Center installed one-way observation windows into the main room from a separate entry hall for just this reason—to allow observers to see the center during daytime hours of operation without distracting residents or making them feel like objects of curiosity. The "quiet week" study discussed earlier also found that staff members or visitors walking *quickly* through the facility were particularly disturbing to residents, who were distracted by this commotion and frequently insisted on knowing "what was going on" or on following these people.

Variability in Tolerance for Stimulation

In addition to variability by personality and source of stimulation, preference or tolerance for social stimulation is also probably related to stage of the disease, as low-functioning residents frequently displayed little tolerance for high levels of social and other stimulation. In an interesting anecdote, staff members at the Alzheimer Care Center noted that a resident who began to spend less time in large-group activities and common spaces and more time in the (less populated and quieter) administrative area was usually the next resident to leave the facility due to progression of the disease.

Desirable amounts of stimulation also vary by time of day for most residents. High-stimulus and high-concentration activities such as group games, dancing, and aerobic exercise are frequently scheduled during typically "high-functioning" morning hours, and low-stimulus activities such as naps, quiet hour, and independent activities frequently take place during the afternoon, when residents typically experience low concentration and high agitation.

The Residential Component

Several questions arise concerning the planning, design, and development of the residential component in environments for people with dementia. Foremost among these are two concerns: (1) the debate over the relative merits of private versus shared rooms and (2) conflicting recommendations concerning cueing of resident rooms, using personalization and things from the past, color, and various types of "signage" to enhance room recognition (Calkins, in press).

Private versus shared resident rooms: pros and cons

Facility planners, regulatory code developers, researchers, facility administrators, and staff members have long argued over the relative merits of private versus shared resident rooms for people with dementia. Proponents of private rooms suggest that single rooms provide privacy and a space for solitary retreat; opportunities for personalization, autonomy, and independence; and a familiar and homelike setting (Cohen and Weisman 1991). Opponents counter that private rooms are unnecessarily expensive and that shared rooms provide important opportunities for social interaction between roommates (Calkins, in press).

Both sides of this debate were reflected in the opinions of administrators and staff members informally surveyed in this research. As expected, staff members in facilities with single rooms tended to favor these, pointing to the benefits of privacy and autonomy so provided. Several newly designed facilities, such as the Corinne Dolan Alzheimer Center in Chardon, Ohio, have only single rooms for residents with dementia, reflecting support of these assumptions. At the same time, those in facilities with shared rooms praised the social interaction encouraged by sharing a room and the absence of resident withdrawal. For example, the administrator and the director of Cedar Lake Home Campus Friendship House reported that, even given sufficient resources to provide all single rooms for their residents, shared rooms were preferred because of the interaction they fostered.

Most interesting were the opinions of staff members and administrators in facilities that provided both shared and private rooms or that had provided both options at some time in the past. Care providers in settings that had experienced both options tended to favor private rooms. For example, the director of the Alzheimer Care Center in Gardiner, Maine, which provides shared rooms for long-term residents and private rooms for respite clients, stated that, given the option, she would prefer all single resident rooms because of the privacy these afford and the usefulness of single rooms as a "quiet space" for agitated residents.

Aside from their therapeutic benefits or detriments, private rooms are often more desirable than shared rooms to family caregivers of residents, who perceive private rooms as more familiar, dignified, and homelike for their family member. For instance, in New Perspective Group Home #4, residents and their caregivers may select from among three room options: shared, private, and private with a personal bathroom. Private rooms with personal bathrooms are 15 percent more expensive than shared rooms with detached bathrooms, yet the former is by far the most requested option. In fact, the New Perspective group home currently under construction will now provide only private rooms with personal bathrooms.

Ensuring flexibility in design—to accommodate both options—is one means of addressing this issue. For example, Minna Murra Lodge in Queensland, Australia, provides all private rooms for its fifteen residents. However, the movable wardrobe that separates single rooms can be rearranged to create one large room for a couple, if desired (fig. 3.16).

An elegant solution providing privacy and autonomy in a double room can be seen in Alexian Village of Milwaukee, Wisconsin. The L-shaped room offers spatial separation and a sense of ownership to each tenant (see chapter 2, "Alexian Village").

Figure 3.16
In this flexible solution, the movable wardrobe serves as a partition between these single rooms. It can be relocated to create a double room for a couple. (Minna Murra Lodge, Toowoomba, Queensland, Australia)

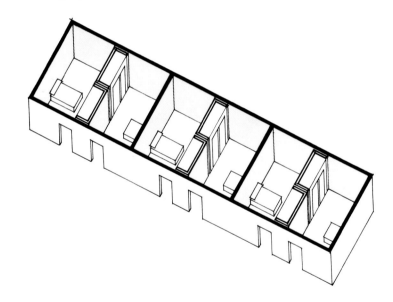

Cueing strategies for increasing recognition of residents' rooms

The second major issue concerns the use of cues and markers to distinguish residents' rooms and to aid residents in identifying their own rooms. Personalization and the incorporation of items from one's previous home is an almost universally accepted strategy; residents are frequently encouraged to bring along a favorite piece of furniture and other personal items with which to furnish and decorate their own rooms. Facility administrators hope that such a policy will not only create less institutional residents' rooms, but also aid residents in identifying their own rooms. Other facilities differentiate residents' rooms on the basis of wallpaper patterns or the color of walls, carpet, curtains, bedspreads, or furnishings. This tactic is intended to serve as an identifying cue for residents, who may be instructed to look for the appropriate color room. (Of course, variety in decoration may be adopted for simple aesthetic

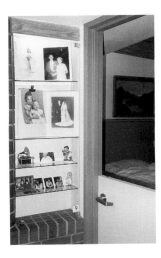

Figure 3.17
Locked glass cabinets filled with a resident's personal belongings serve as an effective aid to identification outside of each resident's room. (Corinne Dolan Alzheimer Center, Chardon, Ohio; photo by Maggie Calkins.)

reasons as well.) Finally, residents' rooms are usually marked with some type of sign, name plate, photograph, or personal momento to aid residents in identification. Although all solutions are probably effective in at least some instances, staff reports regarding the success of various methods of cueing suggest mixed results.

Staff members frequently suggested that, as an identifying device, incorporation of things from the past may be successful for high functioning residents but probably has little effect on moderate- and low-functioning residents. In the design of a new facility to replace the existing Friendship House, facility directors have chosen to eliminate personal furnishings from residents' rooms. While this policy had been helpful for former, high-functioning residents, administrators believe that, given the low functioning levels of the current population, personalization of this kind no longer has any measurable effect either on residents' ability to identify their rooms or on maintenance of links with their pasts.

The same was reported regarding variety in color schemes and furnishings provided by the facility: while this may be effective for high functioning residents as a cue to locate the correct corridor or one's own room, variety in color or wallpaper pattern seems to make little difference to low functioning residents. The director of the Alzheimer Care Center estimates that color cueing by residential wing seems to help about 50 percent of group home residents to locate their own rooms. On the other hand, the director of New Perspective Group Home #4 reports that color cueing is not at all successful as an identification device in this group home; without name signs outside the doors, most residents would never find their rooms.

Interesting discussions centered around the use of various types of door markers or signs to identify each individual resident's room. Every residential facility included in these case studies employed some such marker; these ranged from engraved name plates, to construction paper signs created by staff members, to photographs or personal items outside the door, to full-size glass cabinets filled with a resident's personal momentos. In Stonefield Home, each residential wing is also marked with the names of residents who live on that corridor. In the Alzheimer Care Center, each resident's room is identified with both his or her name and one or more favorite photographs from the past, mounted behind a glass plate to protect the photographs from damage by residents. Pictures from the past were adopted because many residents are unable to identify a current picture of themselves. In most facilities, staff members report that at least some residents seem to be aided by door signs or markers of any form; however, both anecdotal and research evidence supports the hypothesis that personal, meaningful items seem to be most effective in helping residents to locate their own rooms. The doors of residents' room in Friendship House are marked with both signs made by staff members and trinkets attached to the door by family members. Staff members report that the residents with personal trinkets on the door seem to be more effective in locating their rooms. Researchers at the Corinne Dolan Alzheimer Center (Namazi, Rosner, and Rechlin 1991) filled glass display cases outside residents' rooms with both nonmeaningful items and meaningful, personal items of the resident and compared the success of both as identifying devices to help residents to locate their rooms (fig. 3.17). Personal items were demonstrated to be more effective than those that had no personal meaning for residents.

Staying Dry*

Incontinence among people with dementia was a major problem in most of the facilities included in this research, due to both a great number of incontinent people with dementia, and to the early stage in which incontinence often begins. In many cases, the level of incontinence experienced was much higher than facility planners or developers had been led to expect, resulting in significant changes in facility design and operation after admission of the residents. Staff members' and administrators' strategies for dealing with incontinence can be classified into three major types: (1) policy, (2) programmatic, and (3) environmental. Many facilities employed two or three types of strategies concurrently.

Policy-oriented strategies

Policy-oriented strategies for controlling and coping with incontinence emphasized the establishment of criteria for admission and discharge in consideration of the facility's ability to serve incontinent residents. For example, staff members at New Perspective Group Home #4 found, soon after the opening of the facility, that incontinence levels among its residents were much higher than anticipated. Facility planners had originally expected that most residents would be continent; incontinence was expected to factor into the decision to dismiss a resident from the facility. After this realization, New Perspective administrators adopted a conscious policy decision that, given the great number of incontinent residents and the early stages at which incontinence had begun among otherwise competent residents, mild bladder incontinence would not constitute a criteria for refusing admission to the facility.

Administrators at the Alzheimer Care Center in Gardiner, Maine, reached the same conclusion. In addition, they realized that the geriatric evaluation being conducted on all residents before admission did not detect the actual level of incontinence. In response, the evaluation was restructured to include very specific questions regarding incontinence, allowing administrators to identify those residents with more than occasional incidents of incontinence prior to admission.

Program-oriented strategies

Programmatic strategies for controlling incontinence included bowel and bladder examinations of incontinent residents to rule out physical causes (other than AD); adherence to regular (i.e., every two hours) toileting schedules; and diapering of incontinent residents.

The decision to adopt primarily programmatic (rather than environmental)

*This evocative title is borrowed from K. L. Burgio, L. Pearce, and A. J. Lucco (1990). *Staying dry: A practical guide to bladder control.* Baltimore: Johns Hopkins University Press.

strategies may involve consideration of staffing ratios. Elderkare, a group home in Beloit, Wisconsin, was intentionally designed and staffed to accommodate toileting as a programmatic rather than an environmental issue. Each resident in the facility has a private room; however, all residents share three common bathrooms. Facility planners here felt that the addition of a bathroom (with its additional door) to each resident room would confuse residents. In addition, because bathrooms often serve as the site of negative behaviors such as inappropriate voiding, facility planners felt that toileting should be supervised. For these reasons, a decision was made to design the facility for common bathrooms and to adopt a programmatic strategy to control incontinence. Staff members toilet all residents on a regular, two-hour schedule. This strategy is possible at Elderkare because of the high staffing ratio and the fact that each staff member is assigned to care for four individual residents throughout the day and evening. Often, family members resent the absence of private bathrooms, finding common bathrooms institutional. However, most caregivers eventually support this decision, as residents' continence often actually improves upon admission to the facility.

Environmental strategies

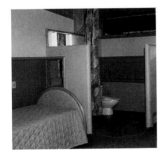

Figure 3.18
Toilets are located in one corner of each resident's room, screened by a curtain when in use. By increasing the visibility of the toilet, facility designers hope to remind residents to visit the bathroom and to increase their ease in locating proper facilities. (Corinne Dolan Alzheimer Center, Chardon, Ohio; photo by Maggie Calkins.)

The decision to adopt environmental strategies (in addition to or instead of the above) is often based on both philosophical and practical grounds. Environmental strategies to control incontinence are frequently intended to preserve the privacy and autonomy of residents. In addition, facilities without intensive staff resources may rely on the physical environment to assist residents in remembering, finding, and using the toilet and to moderate the negative effects of incontinence.

Incontinent residents frequently may not independently remember to use the toilet. The Corinne Dolan Alzheimer Center has adopted an experimental, environmental solution to this problem: in this facility, toilets are placed in the corner of each resident's room, surrounded by five-foot-high partition walls and a curtain for privacy, which is left open when not in use (fig. 3.18). Facility planners hope that the obvious location of the toilet will remind residents to use it when they see it. Research at this facility supports the usefulness of this adaptation. (Of course, this strategy may also help residents to locate the toilet when they are already searching for it.) Administrators in other facilities object to this solution, suggesting that it is unfamiliar and undignified to residents (and that they may not recognize the function of the toilet in this uncommon arrangement).

People with dementia also suffer from wayfinding deficits, resulting in an inability to locate a bathroom when they require one. Facilities that provide private bathrooms attached to residents' rooms suggest that the familiar, residential placement of the bathroom (next to the bedroom) may help residents to locate the toilet. In Stonefield Home, the private bathroom can be seen from the resident's bed, both reminding the resident to use the toilet and helping him or her to locate it easily. Facilities also employ various types of signage to direct residents to bathroom areas and to help them identify bathrooms.

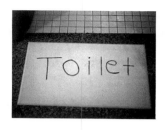

Figure 3.19
Creative staff members devised a special sign on the floor for an incontinent resident who walks with her head lowered. (New Perspective Group Home #4, Mequon, Wisconsin)

St. Ann Day Care Center utilizes international pictograms in the hall outside the bathroom, as well as cueing in the color teal in the area leading up to the bathrooms. Administrators here believe that participants tend to remember color associations longer than written words.

At New Perspective Group Home #4, a special sign was devised to assist one resident who consistently had difficulties in locating the bathroom. Because this resident always walked with her head lowered, she did not notice the prominent signs pointing to the bathroom. Staff printed the word TOILET in large letters on a rubber mat on the floor, where it could be easily seen by the resident; they are not yet certain whether this strategy has resolved the resident's wayfinding problem (fig. 3.19).

Environmental approaches have also been employed to increase ease in using bathroom facilities. Toilet seats at the Alzheimer Care Center are painted a bright color to make the toilet obvious to residents who may otherwise void inappropriately in sinks or waste baskets. All three common bathrooms at Elderkare are wheelchair accessible and equipped for handicapped residents, despite the fact that all residents are ambulatory. Administrators here have found that ambulatory residents also benefit from the extra support of grab bars, as residents with distorted depth perception may be afraid to lower themselves onto toilet seats.

Finally, environmental solutions to problems of sanitation associated with incontinence primarily involved the application of various residential, soil-resistant materials. At Elderkare, living room furnishings are all coated heavily with a spray-on fabric protector. The bottom of each seat is easily removable, to prevent urine pooling. In addition, some chairs are covered with a non-institutional-looking fabric that "feels" like vinyl, as incontinent residents may be ashamed or embarrassed to use fabric-covered chairs that seem damageable, regardless of staff members' assurances to the contrary. At Stonefield Home, one resident room with a tile floor is reserved for an incontinent resident. While practical, this solution may have a stigmatizing or demoralizing effect on that individual.

Family Visiting and Participation

Visiting by friends and family members is an activity that has a range of environmental implications for facilities for people with dementia, many of which may be unexpected. This section explores (1) possible relationships between visiting and design, (2) the use of the environment as a catalyst for interaction, (3) visiting in outdoor environments, and (4) entry areas.

Possible relationships between visiting and design

Many assumptions underlie the design and programming of facilities, activities, and policies to accommodate visiting in environments for people with dementia. Facility planners and administrators assume that "good" design can increase visiting and that visiting is desirable for both residents and caregivers. The design and programming of noninstitutional environments is often recommended at least partially on the premise that these will encourage visiting by family members (Cohen and Weisman 1991). The argument is made that homelike, residential facilities are less distressing and guilt-inducing than institutional settings to family members, who may enjoy visiting more and may consequently visit more frequently when the environment and activities are appealing and familiar. This is particularly important for young children and grandchildren, who may find a domestic environment and "things to do" an added incentive for visiting.

Case study visits offer at least one example where the reverse seems to be true: staff members at the Alzheimer Care Center reported that visiting in their facility seems to be low precisely because the environment and care program are attractive, noninstitutional, and successful. In this boarding home and day care center, visiting occurs most frequently among family members of day care participants and residents who have lived in the facility for less than a year, and visiting tapers off noticeably for longer-time residents. Staff members were initially disappointed at this trend; they had hoped that the cheerful, residential nature of the environment, staff, and activities would encourage family caregivers to participate more frequently than they might in other care options. Another care provider noted that, in day care facilities, staff members would often prefer that families not visit, as this can be disturbing to the family member, staff, and other participants.

A survey of all family members was conducted to ascertain whether caregivers were satisfied with the facility and the type and level of care of residents. Responses were overwhelmingly positive. Caregivers also continued faithfully to attend quarterly conferences at the center and displayed extreme distress if a family member was discharged from the facility. Staff members resolved that families of residents reduce visiting and contact as they go through a process of grieving and acceptance of the realities of the disease. This "letting go" can only occur if caregivers trust that their family member is happy and well cared for in a safe and healthy setting. Staff members hypothesize that, often, visiting in other facilities may be a function of "watchdogging"— efforts by the family member to supervise the care and safety of the resident, monitor chemical and physical restraints and therapy, and ensure the security of personal belongings. Because family members have confidence in the level of care and the nature of the atmosphere of the Alzheimer Care Center, they may feel secure enough to trust the care of their family member to the facility and to begin the necessary process of grieving and acceptance. This realization has prompted staff members here to redefine their goals and objectives in terms of visiting and family participation; while numerous opportunities are still provided for family visiting activities, staff members now accept that participation may be most prevalent among caregivers of day care members and new residents and that the goal of the well-designed, noninstitutional facility may be to instill sufficient confidence in family members to allow them to begin gradually to "let go" of the resident.

This speculation is also supported by the experiences of staff members at Cedar Acres Adult Day Care. Administrators here report that the family of a day care participant becomes as much a client and a responsibility of the facility as the actual participant. Caregivers require significant time and resources from both staff and administration. Administrators hypothesize that family members of day care clients may be particularly dependent because day care is often the first environment or service with which a family will have contact after the diagnosis of Alzheimer's disease. Caregivers of day care participants are frequently in the early stages of shock and coping with the disease and usually have a great need for information, referrals, assistance in financial and medical planning, and other forms of technical and moral support. Cedar Acres has a social worker and even a part-time financial advisor to help caregivers address some of these needs. Many other day care centers (as well as other care environments) also have a support group to help caregivers through this difficult period. The demands of family members even have spatial implications, as the center reported a dire need for a conference room to accommodate frequent meetings and consultations with family members, currently taking place in cramped office quarters.

Administrators at the Alois Alzheimer Center reported that the level of intervention required by a family seems to be directly linked to the way in which a family functions rather than to the type of service provided or the length of experience with Alzheimer services or programs.

Finally, whether the goal of a facility is to encourage visiting by family members or to instill sufficient confidence to allow visiting to decrease, both require the same physical response. An attractive, homelike, and noninstitutional environment is a key ingredient in realizing these goals.

Use of the environment as a catalyst for interaction

Conversation objects and places and equipment for "things to do"—such as games, outdoor gardening areas, and craft centers—were incorporated into the design of some facilities, in part to increase the success and enjoyment of visiting. Such items distributed in areas where visiting occurs provide residents and guests with something to do or talk about when visiting. These things may reduce null or passive behavior on the part of the resident, which may make visiting depressing or frustrating for the guest and discourage further visiting. In addition, such items act as a diversion to family members searching for conversation topics, giving them something to talk about rather than interrogating the resident for details about daily activities, meals, etc., that the resident may not remember. At Friendship House, a giant swordfish hangs in a corner frequently used for visiting with family members. Staff members report that as many people comment negatively as positively about the fish; however, this is the goal of the object—to stimulate conversation—and it accomplishes that objective. Similarly, some old agricultural implements at the outdoor park in Sunset Haven, Ontario, act as a catalyst for reminiscence and conversation.

The opportunity to make a cup of tea or coffee or dish up a bowl of ice cream is a universal ingredient of social interaction. Many facilities, such as the Helen Bader Center, Namesté, New Perspective Group Home #4, St. Ann Day

Center, have serving kitchens and adjoining intimate dining tables, which are accessible and inviting to visitors and residents.

At New Perspective Group Home #4, games and play equipment—including a small basketball and a freestanding hoop—for children are stored in the activity room. In addition to the manifest function of providing "something to do" for visiting children, this equipment also serves the latent function of encouraging children to visit with their parents and providing an activity for visiting families to watch and discuss.

Outdoor areas for visiting

Outdoor areas were reported as especially popular destinations for visiting in several of the facilities discussed. Administrators at the Alzheimer Care Center, Sunset Haven, and Minna Murra Lodge all reported that, although all facilities also offer alternative indoor locations, family members and residents seem to prefer to visit outdoors when weather permits (fig. 3.20). In addition, staff members at numerous facilities, when describing a particularly successful and well-attended family activity, frequently mentioned a picnic, barbecue, or other outdoor event hosted at the facility. Experience at the Alois Alzheimer Center suggests that outings, parties, and celebrations help family members to spend time together without the pressure of one-on-one communication. Although little is known about the specific characteristics of outdoor spaces that encourage this response (but see under "Outdoor Activities" for more information), planners and designers should anticipate and maximize the opportunities for outdoor areas to encourage and sustain visiting activity.

Figure 3.20

The outdoor courtyard is the most popular destination for visiting in Minna Murra Lodge, despite the provision of many alternative indoor activity nooks and social spaces. Family members and residents appreciate the cool breezes, attractive plantings, and familiar, residential nature of this spot. (Minna Murra Lodge, Toowoomba, Queensland, Australia)

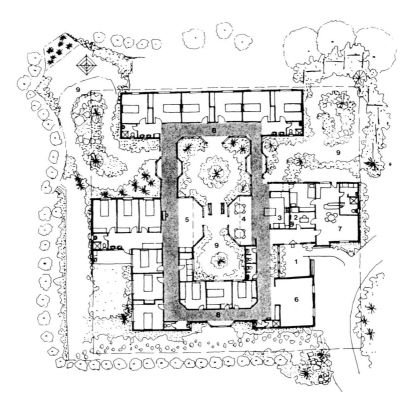

Entrance areas: design potentials and liabilities for visiting

Entrance areas were used in two primary and contrasting ways in regard to visiting. In some facilities, such as St. Ann Day Care Center, the entrance area is conceived and designed as a space for visitors, essentially off-limits to residents. At St. Ann, elegant furnishings and decorations in the entry area present a positive and professional image of the center to visitors and prospective clients and to family members dropping off and picking up participants. The entry hall contains one-way observation windows into the actual activity spaces of the center, eliminating the need to disturb participants with constant visits by architects and program developers interested in the facility. A small room in this entry area is used by students training at the facility; a "guest" restroom is located in this area as well.

Entry areas were also occasionally designed as auxiliary, semipublic social spaces, used for visiting with residents. In Friendship House at Cedar Lake Home Campus in West Bend, Wisconsin, visiting frequently takes place in the ground floor entrance area, one floor beneath the residential households. The designation of this space as a "visiting area" gives residents and their guests "somewhere to go" during visits, both for privacy and as a destination for walks during visits. The environment includes a reception area and a large "living room" with a fireplace. The overall image is of a lobby of a country inn, which in this case includes displays of residents' craft projects and objects from the past to stimulate conversation. Because it is used by residents, the space is decorated in a homelike, informal manner. (However, some staff members disapprove of this design decision, feeling that it presents an unprofessional image of the facility.) Regardless of how the entry area is used and designed with respect to visiting activity, staff members at most facilities recommend that actual entrances be situated out of view and out of the line of traffic of activity areas. Entrances that are clearly visible to wandering residents or from activity areas seem to encourage residents to attempt to leave the facility, either independently or with exiting guests and staff members. This situation causes frustration and agitation (especially if such attempts trigger disruptive alarms) and mandates constant staff supervision and intervention. This may be especially true in day care centers, which experience a great deal of traffic from family members dropping off and picking up participants.

Outdoor Environments

The use of outdoor parks, gardens, patios, and courtyards is relatively neglected in environments for people with dementia. A contributing factor may be the fact that most early special care units were established in skilled nursing facilities, which typically did not provide much of an outdoor extension.

Of the sample of settings described in this book, most facilities have some outdoor activity area. However, few facilities consider the outdoors as an extension of the indoors or as a major activity area integral to the facility program. Noted exceptions include Woodside Place in Oakmont, Pennsylvania; the Corinne Dolan Alzheimer Center in Chardon, Ohio; the Alois Alzheimer

Center in Greenhills, Ohio; and Minna Murra Lodge in Queensland, Australia. The master plan for Pathways continuum of care community in Miami, Florida, also includes extensive outdoor development, from landscaped, protected pedestrian malls to waterways and a lake for caregivers and visitors.

Climate and the feasibility of outdoor development

Temperature and favorable climatic conditions that allow year-round use of the outdoors are certainly a positive incentive to invest in outdoor development. Pathways, in Miami (still in the planning stages), and settings such as Minna Murra Lodge, in Australia, and other facilities in California and Hawaii regard their outdoor environments as important activity areas of significant therapeutic value.

However, it seems that harsher climates in northern states should not be considered an obstacle to outdoor development and use; perhaps *because* of the short, seasonal use of outdoor parks and gardens, these become more valuable to residents and staff members. Most of the northern case study sites included some type of outdoor extension to the facility. In fact, some of the most comprehensive plans for outdoor spaces are located in less-than-tropical regions (e.g., Corinne Dolan Alzheimer Center's outdoor park in Ohio, Woodside Place's series of gardens in Pennsylvania, and several outdoor parks in regional Niagara, Ontario). Conscientious design can maximize the use of outdoor spaces in such places.

Location, access, and spatial relationships

The location and accessibility of the outdoor space and its spatial and conceptual relationship to the facility critically affect the use and success of outdoor environments. A major outdoor park at Sunset Haven, Ontario, is underutilized because of its relative obscurity and inaccessibility. Because of its late development, the 30,000-square foot park was not integrated with the facility building itself. It cannot be seen from public interior spaces, and entry/exit points are remote (see "Therapeutic Garden, Sunset Haven Home for the Aged".

The small, interior courtyard at Stonefield Home is an example of a modest space that functions as an organizing element in the building plan (fig. 3.21). The central courtyard provides light and outdoor views to public interior spaces in all four directions; it is highly accessible—both visually and physically—and well integrated with the building.

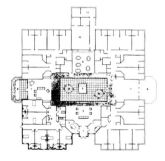

Figure 3.21
The central interior court is an integrated and accessible outdoor space. In addition, two peripheral outdoor spaces serve the neighboring households. (Stonefield Home, Middleton, Wisconsin)

Above-Ground Level Outdoor Space

Information from site visits and interviews suggests that moving residents of units housed in above-ground-level accommodations to ground level outdoor space is complicated, energy consuming, and often disruptive. A possible design response to this problem is the provision of an extensive outdoor extension in the form of a balcony or a terrace, with appropriate features and qualities. This approach is employed by the Helen Bader Center, Milwaukee (now in the planning stages). Another approach is the provision of an indoor atrium or greenhouse, which may include many outdoor features and provide a "surrogate" outdoor experience.

Features that might be included

Some recent designs of facilities demonstrate the potential for comprehensive use and integration of outdoor spaces in the overall plan of the facility. One illustration of an integrated plan with intensive use of the outdoors is Woodside Place, in Oakmont, Pennsylvania (fig. 3.22).

Particular design features

Several design features and qualities of outdoor spaces are now considered common knowledge for designers. These include the use of nontoxic plant materials, the creation of positive microclimates, various shelters from sun and wind, the provision of wheelchair accessibility, and so on.

Further elaboration of microenvironmental design responsive to people with dementia is described in a recent article by Lovering (1990; see also Regnier 1985). Lovering's design of a therapeutic park for Sunset Haven (see "Therapeutic Garden, Sunset Haven") and other design developments include features such as raised planters, bird feeders, and garden swings, all of which provide destinations and landmarks for residents. Rest stops can be accommodated by various seating arrangements. A continuous path supports meaningful wandering. Social interaction, privacy, and appropriate stimulation are all addressed by design and program. Particularly interesting is the use of solutions unique to the outdoors, such as a fragrance garden or a lookout terrace.

Figure 3.22

Individual outdoor courtyards are accessible from each of the households. These sunlit courtyards open to a large, common outdoor area designed for wandering, sitting, and outdoor eating and activities. An additional shared courtyard houses planters for gardening, and the adjacent covered veranda allows the use of the outdoors in more inclement weather. All residents' rooms have visual access to one or more outdoor spaces. (Woodside Place, Oakmont, Pennsylvania; drawing by David Hoglund.)

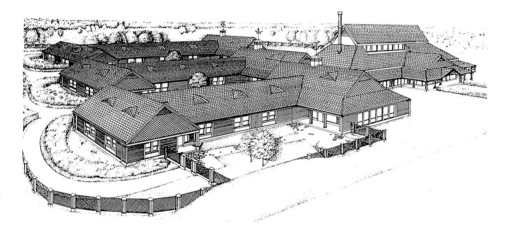

References

Alzheimer's Association (1991). *Public Policy Update.* Chicago: Alzheimer's Association. July.

American National Standards Institute (1980). *Specifications for making buildings and facilities accessible to and usable by physically handicapped people. ANSI 117.1.* New York: American National Standards Association.

Benson, D., Cameron, D., Humbach, E., Servino, L. and Gambert, S. (1987). Establishment and impact of a dementia unit within a nursing home. *American Geriatrics Society, 35* (4), 320–323.

Calkins, M. (1988). *Design for dementia: Planning environments for the elderly and confused.* Owing Mills, Md.: National Health Publishing.

———. (n.d.). Physical environment as a treatment modality. In D. A. Davidoff, H. R. Kessler, and N. Venna (eds.), *Multidisciplinary approaches to the management and treatment of Alzheimer's disease.* Norwell, Mass.: Kluwer Academic Publishers. In press.

Cohen, U., and Weisman, G. (1991). *Holding on to home: Designing environments for people with dementia.* Baltimore: Johns Hopkins University Press.

Coons, D. (1985). Alive and well at Wesley Hall. *Quarterly: A Journal of Long Term Care, 21* (2), 10–14.

——— (1988). Wandering. *American Journal of Alzheimer's Care and Related Disorders and Research, 3* (1), 31–36.

Fraser, D. (1978). Behavioral effects of environmental changes among a psychiatric geriatric population. Pilot Project 2. Norristown State Hospital Psychology Department, Norristown, Pa.

Gilleard, C. (1984). *Living with dementia: Community care of the elderly mentally infirm.* Philadelphia: Charles Press.

Gubrium, J. (1986). *Oldtimers and Alzheimer's disease: The descriptive organization of senility.* Greenwich, Conn.: Jai Press.

Gywther, L. (1986). Treating behavior as a symptom of illness. *Provider,* May, 18–21.

Hall, G., and Buckwalter, K. (1986). *Progressively lowered stress threshold: A conceptual model for care of adults with Alzheimer's disease.* Paper presented at the annual meeting of the American Association of Neurosciences Nurses, 15 April 1986, Denver, Colo.

Harris, D. K. (1988). Dictionary of Gerontology. Westport, Conn.: Greenwood Publishing Group.

Heston, L., and White, J. (1983). *Dementia: A practical guide to Alzheimer's disease and related illnesses.* New York: W. H. Freeman and Co.

Hiatt, L. (1981). Designing therapeutic dining. *Nursing Homes.* April/May, 33–39.

Howell, S. (1980). *Designing for aging: Patterns of use.* Cambridge: MIT Press.

Hyde, J. (1989). The physical environment and the care of Alzheimer's patients: An experiential survey of Massachusetts' Alzheimer's units. *American Journal of Alzheimer's Care and Related Disorders and Research, 4* (3), 36–44.

Kelly, W. (ed.) (1984). *Alzheimer's disease and related disorders. Research and management.* Springfield, Ill.: Charles C. Thomas.

Koncelik, J. (1976). Human factors and environmental design for the aging: Aspects of physiological change and sensory loss as design criteria. In T. Byerts, S. Howell, and L. Pastalan (eds.), *Environmental context of aging* (pp. 107–117). New York: Garland STPM.

Lawton, M. P. (1970). Ecology and aging. In L. Pastalan and D. A. Carson (eds.), *Spatial behavior of older people.* Ann Arbor: Institute of Gerontology, University of Michigan.

———. (1981). Sensory deprivation and the effect of the environment on management of the patient with senile dementia. In N. Miller and G. Cohen (eds.), *Clinical aspects of Alzheimer's disease and senile dementia* (pp. 251–271). New York: Raven Press.

Lawton, M. P., Fulcomer, M., and Kleban, M. (1984). Architecture for the mentally impaired elderly. *Environment and Behavior, 16,* 730–757.

Lawton, M. P., Leibowitz, B., and Chardon, H. (1970). Physical structure and the behavior of senile patients following ward remodeling. *Aging and Human Development, 1,* 231–239.

Lawton, M. P., and Nahemow, L. (1973). Ecology and the aging process. In C. Eisdorfer and M. P. Lawton (eds.), *Psychology of adult development and aging (pp. 619–674). Washington, D.C.: American Psychological Association.*

Liebowitz, B., Lawton, M. P., and Waldman, A. (1979). Evaluation: Designing for confused elderly people. *American Institute of Architects Journal, 68,* 59–61.

Lindeman, D. (1984). *Alzheimer's disease handbook.* San Francisco: Aging Health Policy Center. Grant No. 90-AP0003.

Lovering, M. J. (1990). Alzheimer's disease and outdoor space: Issues in environmental design. *American Journal of Alzheimer's Care and Related Disorders and Research,* May/June, 33–40.

Mace, N. (1987). Programs and services which specialize in the care of persons with dementing illnesses—issues and options. *American Journal of Alzheimer's Care and Related Disorders and Research,* May/June, 10–17.

Mace, N., and Rabins, P. (1981). *The 36 hour day.* Baltimore: Johns Hopkins University Press.

Mathew, L., Sloan, P., Kilby, M., and Flood, R. (1988). What's different about a special care unit for dementia patients? A comparative study. *American Journal of Alzheimer's Care and Related Disorders and Research,* March/April, 16–23.

Namazi, K. H., Rosner, T. T., and Rechlin, L. R. (1991). Long term memory cuing to reduce visual-spatial disorganization in Alzheimer's disease patients in special care unit. *American Journal of Alzheimer's care and related disorders research, 6*(6), 10–16.

Ohta, R., and Ohta, B. (1988). Special care units for Alzheimer's disease patients: A critical look. *Gerontologist, 28* (6), 803–808.

Pastalan, L. (1979). Sensory changes and environmental behaviors. In T. Byerts, S. Howell, and L. Pastalan (eds.), *Environmental context of aging* (pp. 118–126). New York: Garland STPM.

———. (1990). *Aging in place. The role of housing and social supports.* Binghampton, England: Haworth Press.

Peppard, N. (1986). Effective design of special care units. *Provider*, May, 14–17.

Rapelje, D. H., and Crawford, L. (1987). Creating lively park-spaces for mentally frail seniors in long term care. *Recreation Canada*, December, 23–27.

Rapelje, D. G., Papp, P. P., and Crawford, L. (1981). Creating a therapeutic park for the mentally frail. *Dimensions in health service*, September, 12–14.

Regnier, V. (1985). *Behavioral and environmental aspects of outdoor space use in housing for the elderly.* Los Angeles: Andrus Gerontology Center.

Reisberg, B. (1983). An overview of current concepts of Alzheimer's disease, senile dementia, and age-associated cognitive decline. In B. Reisberg (ed.), *Alzheimer's disease: The standard reference* (pp. 6–20). New York: Free Press.

Roach, M. (1984). Reflections in a fake mirror. *Discover, 8*, 76–85.

Shamoian, C. (1984). *Biology and treatment of dementia in the elderly.* Washington, D.C.: American Psychiatric Press.

Snyder, L. (1984). Archetypal place and the needs of the aging. In M. Spivak (ed.), *Institutional settings: An environmental design approach.* New York: Plenum Press.

Stevens, P. S. (1987). Design for dementia: Recreating the loving family. *American Journal of Alzheimer's Care and Research*, January/February, 16–22.

U.S. Congress Office of Technology Assessment (1987). *Losing a million minds: Confronting the tragedy of Alzheimer's disease and other dementias.* OTA-BA-323. Washington, D.C.: U.S. Government Printing Office.

Index